THE ULTIMATE GUIDE TO
FINDING THE RIGHT JOB AFTER RESIDENCY

THE ULTIMATE GUIDE TO
FINDING THE
RIGHT JOB
AFTER
RESIDENCY

Koushik K. Shaw, MD
Clinical Instructor
Department of Urology
Tulane University School of Medicine
New Orleans, Louisiana
Chief, Section of Urology
Austin Diagnostic Clinic
Austin, Texas

Joyesh K. Raj, MD
Attending Surgeon
Division of Plastic and Reconstructive Surgery
Department of Surgery
Fairview Hospital
Cleveland Clinic Health System
Cleveland, Ohio

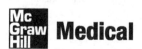 **Medical**

New York   Chicago   San Francisco   Lisbon   London   Madrid   Mexico City   Milan
New Delhi   San Juan   Seoul   Singapore   Sydney   Toronto

The Ultimate Guide to Finding the Right Job after Residency

5 6 7 8 9 0   DOH/DOH   14 13 12 11
ISBN: 0-07-146113-2

Notice

Medicine is an ever-changing science. As new research and clinical experience broaden our knowledge, changes in treatment and drug therapy are required. The authors and the publisher of this work have checked with sources believed to be reliable in their efforts to provide information that is complete and generally in accord with the standards accepted at the time of publication. However, in view of the possibility of human error or changes in medical sciences, neither the authors nor the publisher nor any other party who has been involved in the preparation or publication of this work warrants that the information contained herein is in every respect accurate or complete, and they disclaim all responsibility for any errors or omissions or for the results obtained from use of the information contained in this work. Readers are encouraged to confirm the information contained herein with other sources. For example and in particular, readers are advised to check the product information sheet included in the package of each drug they plan to administer to be certain that the information contained in this work is accurate and that changes have not been made in the recommended dose or in the contraindications for administration. This recommendation is of particular importance in connection with new or infrequently used drugs.

The editors are Catherine A. Johnson and Karen Davis.
The production supervisor was Catherine Saggese.
This book was set in Electra LH by International Typesetting and Composition.
The cover designer was Kelly Parr.
The text designer was Marsha Cohen/Parallelogram Graphics.
The index was prepared by Robert Swanson
RR Donnelley was printer and binder.

This book is printed on acid-free paper.

Library of Congress Cataloging-in-Publication Data

Shaw, Kousik K.
   The ultimate guide to finding the right job after residency / Koushik K. Shaw.
      p. ; cm.
   Includes index.
   ISBN 0-07-146113-2
   1. Physicians–Employment. 2. Job hunting. I. Title
R690.S46 2005
610.69—dc22   2005052204

To my beloved parents, Shyamali and Dilip

Without the strength, encouragement, and love they've provided me over the years, I could never have come so far and achieved what I have in life. This book is a reflection of the virtues of dedication and perseverance you've given to us.

Mom, this one's for you.

Contents

Preface ix

Acknowledgments xi

1. Planning Your Career Search 1

2. Who are You? Profiling the Candidate 3
   Common Pitfalls 16

3. Where Do You Want to Work? Finding the Ideal Practice . 23
   Solo Practice 23
   Joining a Solo Practice 25
   Joining a Single Specialty, Small Group Practice 27
   Single Specialty, Large Group Practice 29
   Joining a Multispecialty Group Practice 31
   Academic Practice 32
   Locum Tenens (Flexible Contracts Involving Varying
      Duration and Geography) 36
   Government (Veterans Affairs, Public Service, etc.) 36

4. The Curriculum Vitae 37

5. Starting Your Search 47
   Locating Leads 47
   Recruiters 49
   Pitfalls 51

6. Preparing for the Interview 53
   Interview Questions 54
   Preparing Answers 55
   Work Surroundings 60
   Financial Analysis 61

7. Understanding Salary and Compensation Arrangements . . 63
   Physician Recruitment Agreements 64
   Compensation Based on Productivity 70

Compensation Based on Group or Physician Net Income ...   70
Formula-Based Compensation   71
Fixed Salary   71
Relative Value Unit-Based Salary   72
Bonuses   72
Special Considerations for Those Considering a Career
  in Academia   73
Note on Ancillary Revenue Streams   74
Overview of Expense Structure   75

8. **Financial Due Diligence: Investigating the Practice**   77

9. **Negotiating a Fair and Proper Contract**   83
Part I: Compensation   86
Part II: Terms of Employment   93
Part III: Termination   98

10. **The Credentialing Process**   103

11. **An Overview of Solo Practice Setup**   107
Solo Practice Considerations   107
Getting Started (1 Year Ahead)   108
Getting Serious (9 Months Ahead)   109
Establishing Benefits and Insurance (6 Months Ahead)   110
Designing and Outfitting Your Practice (6 Months Ahead)   111
Contracting with Insurers (4 Months Ahead)   112
Assembling Your Team (3 Months Ahead)   114
The Final Details (1 to 2 Months Ahead)   114
Almost There! (The Weeks Ahead)   115

12. **Basic Practice Finance 101**   117

Appendix 1. Resources   121

Appendix 2. Physician Compensation Guide   127

Appendix 3. Physician Compensation and Benefits Worksheet   129

Index   133

Preface

It is said that necessity is the mother of invention. Well, the inspiration for this book was born from my recent experience in trying to find the ideal career for myself upon finishing residency. Like most residents and fellows, I was faced with several career decisions. As a member of over 25,000 medical and surgical residents graduating each year, I was surprised to find that no single, comprehensive source of information existed to help with career planning after residency. Instead, I found myself asking a lot of folks about their opinions and thoughts, and occasionally came across a few facts. So, once I found my "ideal" career track, I decided to incorporate a lot of those facts, and a few opinions, into what I hope will be an insightful guide for those young physicians about to tread down a path, leading to the start of a wonderful continuation in the practice of medicine.

It is well known that physicians, especially new graduates, are not always adept in financial planning and management, contract negotiations, legal matters, and such. Unfortunately, it is not the objective of residency programs to educate their young trainees to become "business savvy." I find that young residents find themselves well educated in the art of being a physician, yet in truth, a vast majority find themselves in the position of negotiating the type of practice arrangement, finances, and significant legal issues without an adequate knowledge base. The results can often be disastrous for many who find themselves in contracts or practice groups that do not look after their best interests. This can leave the young physician in further debt and/or a bad practice situation that they did not expect. In fact, of newly graduating physicians, nearly *fifty percent* leave their first job within 2–3 years. I'm left wondering what we're not doing right.

During my own journey through the post residency placement experience, I found that many residents often ask informal networks of friends, family, and older physician/colleagues to help them through the job search process. While recruiters are readily available, they are often driven by other incentives. For example, commissions on the average of 20–40 thousand dollars per recruit means that their best interests may not always be in line with that of a young physician.

As one enters his or her last year of residency, critical questions loom. What defines a solo practice, a single-specialty group, a multi-specialty group, or an academic center? What are the advantages of each? What is an acceptable salary in each of these categories, by region? What are non-compete clauses? Which ones are fair, and which ones can be upheld by law depending on the state you practice in? What items are reasonable to negotiate and what are some tips in negotiating? What is an acceptable "buy-in" to a practice, and what is an acceptable time to partnership? What other intangibles should one look for when interviewing with various practices? What are some red flags to watch for?

I received answers to these and many other questions in the course of my own search, and via a multitude of sources. However, the answers were not always easy to find, and often varied depending on what I read or to whom I spoke. This led to the idea for writing a guide-book which would serve as a single, concise source for young physicians, as well as those physicians who are restarting their job-search in mid-career.

I invite you to share your comments and suggestions for improvement in the next edition of this book. Please send them to:

guidebook@koushikshawmd.com

Koushik K. Shaw, MD
New Orleans, Louisiana
August 2005

Acknowledgments

I would like to acknowledge the contributions of those who made this book possible:

My sister, who exhibits a strength, passion, and excitement in everything she does. She truly is an inspiration to everyone who has had the privilege of having Mousumi in their life, including myself. I am proud to call her my best friend.

My Chairman, for there is only one Raju Thomas (Thank God!). Not only my Chairman, but my mentor and friend as well. He has commanded my respect and admiration from day one, when I had the honor to be recruited to his program. His seemingly boundless energy, strength, and positive energy even in the most challenging of days never ceases to amaze me. I thank him for giving me the skills to be the physician and surgeon I am today. To him, I am eternally grateful.

And finally, the wonderful people of the City of New Orleans. My home for a wonderful period in my life, and in my heart forever. The people I helped as I grew as a physician in training helped me grow as a person. To all of them, I am forever indebted.

1

PLANNING YOUR CAREER SEARCH

One of the first big questions I had when starting my own job search was, "How early is too early?" After asking various recruiters, independent physicians, medical groups, and hospitals, it became evident that it was acceptable, if not highly recommended, that you should start this important process at least *1 year* prior to the anticipated start date. This usually translates to the beginning of the last year of residency (ie, July). Various factors, such as having a general idea of practice location and type of practice, could lengthen or shorten the timetable.

The final year of residency is often a big one, with many professional demands on your time. The best advice is that you *make time* and integrate the search process into your schedule. The latest statistics show that a new physician only stays with his or her first job for about 3 *years.* So, the more time you have on your side, the more time you'll have to dodge the *inevitable* curveballs that will be tossed your way, and thus you will be able to pave a smooth transition to your new practice.

Let's use a July-to-June timeframe (1-year period) to sketch out a rough draft of a timetable; you may want to use it as a guideline to construct your own personalized version.

July	Personal assessment period (self-profiling of candidate, spouse, location, practice type, etc)
August	Initiate search process based on multiple sources and criteria
September	Narrow search based on criteria from self-profile
October	Begin initial set of interviews
November	Continue interview process
December	Continue interview process
January	Start Federal/State credentialing process *(may take up to 6 months to receive licensure and subsequently become a provider on insurance plans)* Evaluate/compare/rank interview sites
February	Second-look interviews
March	Review contracts/legal consultation Follow up on credentialing process
April	Decision process/sign contract
May	Follow up on Federal/State credentialing process Look into debt consolidation services for repayment *(finance rates are reset on July 1st of every year)*
June	Hospital/insurance credentialing and privileges Coordination of move Enjoy a worry-free graduation!

2

WHO ARE YOU?
PROFILING
THE CANDIDATE

Let's start the candidate profile with an evaluation of marital and family status. Being single can often afford you certain more options in terms of geography. Simply put, it may allow you to look at any region of the country you want, depending on your own interests. You may want to balance this with a need to be near family and friends. Or, depending on your needs, you may want to consider more cosmopolitan areas where there will be a higher likelihood of meeting people who share your interests. You may want to refer to the included tables for a ranking of cities with various characteristics (see Tables 1, 2, and 3).

Alternatively, many job opportunities (often, those with higher incomes and salaries) present themselves in small and moderately dense, rural populations. If you're one of the adventurous, independent, outdoors types, willing to "go it on your own" and try your hand in a smaller locale with its intrinsic benefits, you may indeed find many beautiful smaller communities that suit your needs.

Married? Well, as marriage entails compromise, so does the job search process. Depending on your life stage, planning can be as "simple" as coordinating your needs with that of your spouse, or as complex as including additional factors such as availability of quality public and private schooling, special needs education, and family support. Several studies show that living within a one- to two-hour commute of the spouse's family can greatly help the family dynamic. This may be quite important for those with young children or those expecting to start a

TABLE 1

TOP OVERALL CITIES (Based on Nine Categories—Including Economy and Jobs, Cost of Living, Climate, Education, Arts and Culture per Forbes.Com)

THE CITIES

1. Charlottesville, VA
2. Santa Fe, NM
3. San Luis Obispo-Paso Robles, CA
4. Santa Barbara,
5. Honolulu, HI
6. Ann Arbor, MI
7. Atlanta, GA
8. Asheville, NC
9. Reno, NV
10. Corvallis, OR
11. Roanoke, VA
12. Portland-Vancouver,
13. Raleigh-Durham-
14. Bryan-College
15. Lynchburg, VA
16. Olympia, WA
17. Norfolk-Virginia
18. Colorado Springs,
19. Nassau-Suffolk,
20. Pueblo, CO
21. Eugene-Springfield, OR
22. Austin-San Marcos, TX
23. Lafayette, IN
24. Minneapolis-St. Paul, MN
25. Dover, DE
26. Washington, DC-MD-VA-WV
27. Fayetteville-Springdale, AR
28. Pittsburgh, PA
29. Bloomington, IN
30. Stamford-Norwalk, CT
31. State College, PA
32. Abilene, TX
33. Champaign-Urbana, IL
34. Athens, GA
35. Wichita, KS
36. Fort Worth-Arlington, TX
37. Madison, WI
38. Bellingham, WA
39. Las Cruces, NM
40. New York, NY

TABLE 2

TOP CITIES (Based On Nightlife, Culture, Job Growth, Number of Other Singles, and Cost of Living)

THE CITIES

1. Denver-Boulder, Co
2. Washington-Baltimore, DC-MD
3. Austin, TX
4. Atlanta, GA
5. Boston, MA
6. Los Angeles, CA
7. Phoenix, AR
8. New York, NY
9. San Francisco, CA
10. Miami, FL
11. Chicago, IL
12. Dallas-Fort Worth, TX
13. San Diego, Ca.
14. Minneapolis-St Paul, MN
15. Philadelphia, PA
16. Houston, TX
17. Raleigh-Durham, NC
18. Seattle, WA
19. New Orleans, LA
20. Orlando, FL
21. Columbus, OH
22. St. Louis, MO
23. Milwaukee, WI
24. Portland, OR
25. Tampa, FL
26. Las Vegas, NV
27. Indianapolis, IN
28. San Antonio, TX
29. Nashville, TN
30. Kansas City, MO
31. Sacramento, CA
32. Detroit, MI
33. Cleveland, OH
34. Salt Lake City, UT
35. Providence, RI
36. Charlotte, NC
37. Greensboro, NC
38. Norfolk, VA
39. Cincinnati, OH
40. Pittsburgh, PA

TABLE 3

AVERAGE COST* OF A FOUR BEDROOM, 2,200 SQ FT HOME (2004)

Market	Avg Sales Price
Alabama	
Mobile	$180,000
Huntsville	$190,000
Alaska	
Anchorage	$250,000
Juneau	$420,000
Arizona	
Tucson	$220,000
Mesa	$215,000
Phoenix	$270,000
Flagstaff	$330,000
Scottsdale	$380,000
Arkansas	
Fort Smith	$165,000
Little Rock	$170,000
Fayetteville	$210,000
California	
Fresno	$305,000
Bakersfield	$315,000
Modesto	$340,000
Sacramento	$350,000
Riverside/Ontario	$360,000
Grass Valley	$360,000
Palm Desert	$400,000
Santa Clarita	$500,000
Davis	$600,000
San Diego	$610,000
Napa	$640,000
Rancho Bernardo	$650,000
Fullerton	$665,000
Thousand Oaks	$670,000
Santa Rosa	$675,000
Encinitas	$700,000
Walnut Creek	$715,000
Pasadena	$715,000
Monterey Peninsula	$740,000
San Rafael	$740,000
Irvine	$760,000

TABLE 3

AVERAGE COST* OF A FOUR BEDROOM, 2,200 SQ FT HOME (2004) (*CONTINUED*)

MARKET	AVG SALES PRICE
Mission Viejo	$760,000
Pleasanton	$780,000
Fremont	$790,000
Santa Cruz	$790,000
Long Beach	$840,000
San Jose	$950,000
Oakland/Montclair	$960,000
Palos Verdes	$980,000
Santa Monica	$1,100,000
San Francisco	$1,125,000
San Mateo	$1,142,000
Newport Beach	$1,174,000
Palo Alto	$1,212,000
Santa Barbara	$1,230,000
Beverly Hills	$1,313,000
La Jolla	$1,708,000
Colorado	
Colorado Springs	$180,000
Denver	$249,000
Fort Collins	$264,000
Highlands Ranch	$327,000
Boulder	$441,000
Connecticut	
Litchfield County/Torrington	$220,000
Naugatuck	$333,000
Danbury	$365,000
Norwalk	$548,000
Ridgefield	$666,000
Stamford	$681,000
Westport	$753,000
New Canaan	$1,081,000
Westport	$753,000
Greenwich	$1,192,000
Delaware	
Wilmington	$348,000
Florida	
Pensacola	$169,000
Northwest/Panama City	$204,000

(Continued)

TABLE 3

AVERAGE COST* OF A FOUR BEDROOM, 2,200 SQ FT HOME (2004) (*CONTINUED*)

Market	Avg Sales Price
Florida (*Continued*)	
Port Charlotte	$227,000
Gainesville	$228,000
Orlando	$244,000
Tallahassee	$245,000
Tampa	$247,000
Jacksonville	$267,000
Fort Myers	$274,000
Sarasota	$279,000
Daytona Beach	$291,000
Boca Raton	$304,000
Clearwater/St. Petersburg	$310,000
Fort Lauderdale/Coral Springs	$323,000
West Palm Beach	$323,000
Naples	$346,000
Miami/Coral Gables	$507,000
Key West	$759,000
Georgia	
Dalton	$172,000
Macon	$178,000
Columbus	$207,000
Athens	$221,000
Savannah	$239,000
Atlanta	$283,000
Hawaii	
Kihei, Maui	$591,000
Honolulu	$614,000
Kailua, Kona	$1,087,000
Idaho	
Coeur d'Alene	$180,000
Boise	$192,000
Illinois	
Springfield	$168,000
Rockford	$179,000
Peoria	$203,000
Bloomington	$206,000
Champaign	$218,000
Joliet	$225,000
Elgin	$257,000

TABLE 3

AVERAGE COST* OF A FOUR BEDROOM, 2,200 SQ FT HOME (2004) (*CONTINUED*)

MARKET	AVG SALES PRICE
Flossmoor	$272,000
Aurora	$275,000
Orland Park	$308,000
Schaumburg	$309,000
Naperville	$322,000
Carol Stream	$333,000
Deerfield	$510,000
Barrington	$530,000
Chicago	$763,000
Indiana	
Evansville	$166,000
South Bend	$171,000
Fort Wayne	$183,000
Indianapolis	$189,000
Valparaiso	$222,000
Schererville	$235,000
Munster	$299,000
Iowa	
Dubuque	$177,000
Cedar Rapids	$107,000
Sioux City	$227,000
Des Moines	$242,000
Kansas	
Topeka/Shawnee County	$141,000
Wichita/Sedgwick County	$154,000
Leavenworth/Lansing	$189,000
Overland Park	$206,000
Lawrence	$226,000
Kentucky	
Lexington	$155,000
Northern Kentucky/Florence	$196,000
Louisville	$223,000
Louisiana	
Lafayette	$171,000
Baton Rouge	$197,000
Shreveport/Bossier City	$214,000
New Orleans	$250,000

(Continued)

TABLE 3

AVERAGE COST* OF A FOUR BEDROOM, 2,200 SQ FT HOME (2004) (*CONTINUED*)

MARKET	AVG SALES PRICE
Maine	
Lewiston/Auburn	$166,000
Augusta	$195,000
Bangor	$213,000
Portland	$334,000
Maryland	
Eastern Shore	$247,000
Hagerstown/Washington County	$270,000
Westminster/Carroll County	$293,000
Metro Baltimore	$293,000
Bel Air/Harford County	$296,000
Waldorf/Charles County	$296,000
Annapolis/Anne Arundel County	$337,000
Frederick	$338,000
Columbia/Howard County	$391,000
Bethesda/Chevy Chase/Montgomery County	$491,000
Massachusetts	
Greater Springfield	$291,000
Worcester	$311,000
Taunton	$411,000
Framingham	$509,000
Barnstable/Cape Cod	$548,000
Acton	$700,000
Lexington	$715,000
Boston	$1,053,000
Wellesley	$1,102,500
Michigan	
Cadillac	$145,000
Gaylord	$171,000
Grayling/Roscommon	$189,000
Mt. Pleasant	$199,000
Grand Rapids	$199,000
Midland/Saginaw/Bay City	$219,000
Port Huron	$219,000
Jackson	$236,000
Flint Metro/Grand Blanc	$237,000
Petoskey	$239,000
Greater Lansing	$240,000
Auburn Hills/Lake Orion	$260,000

TABLE 3

AVERAGE COST* OF A FOUR BEDROOM, 2,200 SQ FT HOME (2004) (*CONTINUED*)

MARKET	AVG SALES PRICE
Indian River	$278,000
Detroit Metro	$282,000
Ann Arbor	$340,000
Traverse City	$229,000
Minnesota	
Moorhead/Clay County	$167,000
Rochester	$208,000
St. Cloud	$229,000
Duluth	$270,000
St. Paul	$346,000
Minneapolis	$354,000
Edina	$367,000
Mississippi	
Tupelo	$166,000
Gulfport/Biloxi	$166,000
Jackson	$219,000
Missouri	
Springfield	$159,000
Kansas City	$201,000
St Louis	$229,000
Montana	
Great Falls	$130,000
Billings	$134,000
Helena	$158,000
Kalispell	$159,000
Bozeman	$256,000
Nebraska	
Omaha	$169,000
North Platte	$173,000
Kearney	$177,000
Nevada	
Las Vegas	$263,000
Reno/Sparks	$347,000
New Hampshire	
Portsmouth	$277,000
Amherst	$296,000
Hanover	$469,000

(Continued)

TABLE 3

AVERAGE COST* OF A FOUR BEDROOM, 2,200 SQ FT HOME (2004) (*CONTINUED*)

Market	Avg Sales Price
New Jersey	
Turnersville/Gloucester County	$231,000
Camden County/Cherry Hill	$257,000
Atlantic County/Absecon	$299,000
Ocean County/Toms River	$332,000
Metuchen/Edison	$421,000
Marlboro/Manalapan	$461,000
Wayne	$501,000
Clinton	$514,000
Sparta	$521,000
Princeton Junction	$559,000
Montclair	$583,000
Madison	$603,000
Basking Ridge	$603,000
Westfield	$672,000
Ridgewood	$752,000
Warren	$753,000
Bridgewater	$525,000
New Mexico	
Albuquerque	$228,000
Santa Fe	$448,000
New York	
Binghamton	$147,000
Syracuse	$205,000
Buffalo	$228,000
Rochester/SE Suburbs	$251,000
Albany	$258,000
Orange County	$338,000
Yorktown Heights	$451,000
Staten Island	$520,000
Long Island	$567,000
Briarcliff Manor	$594,000
Queens (Bayside)	$641,000
North Carolina	
Greensboro	$178,000
Fayetteville	$183,000
Charlotte	$190,000
Winston-Salem	$190,000
Raleigh	$218,000
Wilmington	$229,000

TABLE 3

AVERAGE COST* OF A FOUR BEDROOM, 2,200 SQ FT HOME (2004) (*CONTINUED*)

MARKET	AVG SALES PRICE
North Dakota	
Minot	$130,000
Bismarck	$163,000
Fargo	$184,000
Ohio	
Dayton	$166,000
Akron	$176,000
Toledo	$180,000
Canton	$184,000
Greater Cleveland	$217,000
Columbus	$231,000
Harrison	$202,000
Cincinnati	$234,000
Oklahoma	
Tulsa	$138,000
Oklahoma City	$182,000
Oregon	
Salem	$225,000
Portland	$262,000
Eugene	$265,000
Medford	$317,000
Bend	$319,000
Pennsylvania	
Erie	$183,000
Reading	$216,000
Harrisburg	$228,000
Stroudsburg/Poconos	$229,000
Lancaster	$239,000
York	$239,000
Pittsburgh	$243,000
Allentown	$304,000
Westchester/Chester County	$347,000
Delaware County/Media	$372,000
Doylestown/Bucks County	$392,000
Montgomery County/Conshohocken	$431,000
Philadelphia County/Center City Philadelphia	$488,000
Puerto Rico	
Puerto Rico	$269,000

(Continued)

TABLE 3

AVERAGE COST* OF A FOUR BEDROOM, 2,200 SQ FT HOME (2004) (*CONTINUED*)

Market	Avg Sales Price
Rhode Island	
Providence	$440,000
South Carolina	
Columbia	$175,000
Greenville	$185,000
Myrtle Beach	$187,000
Charleston	$290,000
South Dakota	
Aberdeen	$148,000
Yankton	$149,000
Sioux Falls	$164,000
Rapid City	$174,000
Tennessee	
Knoxville	$145,000
Memphis	$176,000
Chattanooga	$180,000
Nashville	$198,000
Texas	
Arlington	$134,000
Killeen	$136,000
Fort Worth	$148,000
Lubbock	$166,000
Corpus Christi	$168,000
Houston	$173,000
Amarillo	$174,000
El Paso	$174,000
Bryan-College Station	$182,000
Plano	$182,000
Austin	$202,000
San Antonio	$205,000
Dallas	$236,000
Utah	
Provo	$207,000
Salt Lake City	$238,000
Vermont	
Montpelier	$241,000
Rutland	$267,000
Burlington	$279,000

TABLE 3

AVERAGE COST* OF A FOUR BEDROOM, 2,200 SQ FT HOME (2004) (*CONTINUED*)

MARKET	AVG SALES PRICE
Virginia	
Roanoke/Blacksburg	$206,000
Lynchburg	$207,000
Norfolk/Virginia Beach	$223,000
Winchester/Frederick	$244,000
Richmond	$244,000
Lake Ridge/Prince William County	$318,000
Leesburg/Loudoun County	$356,000
Manassas/Prince William County	$368,000
Reston/Fairfax County	$462,000
Alexandria City	$548,000
McLean/Fairfax County	$558,000
Washington	
Spokane	$207,000
Tri-Cities	$225,000
Tacoma	$255,000
Seattle	$341,000
Bellevue	$491,000
Wisconsin	
Eau Claire	$161,000
Wausau	$198,000
Fond du lac	$207,000
Madison	$248,000
Fox Cities	$249,000
Green Bay	$263,000
Milwaukee	$310,000
West Virginia	
Parkersburg	$144,000
Beckley	$156,000
Charleston	$195,000
Wyoming	
Cheyenne	$194,000

*Overall average sales price is $354,372.

Sources: U.S. Census Bureau, U.S. Department of Housing and Development, National Association of Realtors, 2004.

family, especially considering the significant time demands that are needed of the physician joining a new practice.

Two-physician families will need additional planning that requires finding a medical community that will support both specialties and provide for future professional growth. Those with spouses in the technology, legal, or other specialty areas will need to look for cities that have a solid economic and industrial base for these positions. Remember having large corporations and a strong economic base is good for your patient population as well.

"Show me the money" (or lack thereof!). It's hard to ignore finances, and your career choice will significantly affect, and be affected by, your particular financial picture. On average, young physicians will have accumulated significant debt—somewhere between $100,000 and $200,000. You must also take into consideration such factors as being single versus married, and having children. These special factors and others will affect your capacity for debt repayment. The choice of city in which to practice will also have a significant impact upon this ability to survive financially. Remember, that it is not what you earn that is as important as is what you actually "keep" at the end of the day.

Unfortunately, there is often a strong negative correlation between the cost of living and salary ranges across most of the United States. For example, San Diego, with a high cost of living, also has significant competitive forces in play, including managed care penetration, which can drive overall salaries down. Ultimately, the physician receives a financial double "whammy" in the form of low income and high expenses. Conversely, rural areas tend to have less competition than urban areas and higher reimbursements, as well as a lower cost of living. As will be detailed later, these practice situations may be more willing to negotiate debt repayment as part of your contract. So, depending on your unique financial circumstances, choice of location can play a major role in your decision-making process. Refer to Tables 1, 2, and 3 for a detailed comparison of various major cities.

COMMON PITFALLS

When attempting to find the ideal location to fit your personality, lifestyle, and goals, it is important to incorporate both short-term as well as long-term goals. Several mistakes that commonly are made revolve around sacrificing your long-term goals for "what looks good now." Although these decisions may make sense initially, consider the long-term downside of relocation, building, and then rebuilding professional and personal relationships. To this, add the possibility of having to reestablish a patient base and the possibility of expensive contract buy-outs and disputes. Quite simply, it's just not worth it. Although most physicians these days will not stay at one position for the duration of their careers, minimizing career shifts are preferred for obvious reasons.

A common mistake is to "go for the money." Most residents earn between $30,000 and $40,000; combine this with medical school debt that is on average well over $100,000, and it is often tempting to seek out positions that offer starting salaries that are significantly higher than the norm. More often than not, these positions interestingly seem to find you. What do I mean? Well, these are often the offers that are the subject of mailings, cold-calling from recruiters, etc. As in life, where nothing is free, these exorbitant offers often have "hooks," including extended contract periods, large buyout penalties, and troubled backgrounds that experience high turnover. (These contract issues are covered later in the book.)

In addition to this, it is important to distinguish *salary* from your *income*. *Salary* is the up-front dollar figure, or wages paid on a regular basis, where *income* refers to your salary plus any incentives, bonuses, insurance, and ancillary revenue streams. Some positions may offer less up front, but instead offer incentive plans and other benefits, such as health insurance and retirement plans, which over time can end up being a better deal.

In short, it is highly recommended to systematically examine your personal life situation and to incorporate both your long- and short-term goals in identifying your ideal practice location and type.

Examine Tables 1, 2, and 3 and utilize the recommended Web site tools to fill out your personalized list of top cities. After a while, you will begin to see that certain cities and, most importantly, *parts of the country* will appear consistently more often than others. These areas will be referred to later in the book as the discussion on the decision-making process is continued. And a special mention about the rank lists—that they are exactly that (lists) and can vary from source to source and from whom you ask. In fact, your list will be different depending on who you are and what you practice. For instance, if you happen to be an expert in the field of bariatrics, you will be glad to know that Houston, Texas, has been at the top of the list of "fattest" cities, 2 years in a row.

So go ahead, have some fun, read the included rank lists, find your own on the recommended Web sites, and create your individualized ranking of top cities.

One last note: make sure that you include your spouse or significant other, family, friends, and colleagues in this process!

USEFUL WEB SITES

- Salary.com's Cost of Living
  Wizard at http://costoflivingwizard.salary.com. Compare your current location's cost of living to your new location.
- CNN/Money: http://money.cnn.com/real_estate/best_places/ An excellent site that shows full details including education, tax rates crime statistics, and much more on most American cities.
- Sperling's Best Places: http://www.bestplaces.net/fybp/ Great site for comparing statistics on two cities of your choosing, or defining your ideal place to live by ranking various categories. The site will generate a list of cities based on your preferences.
- Crime Statistics: http://www.relocationessentials.com/tools/crime/ crime.asp. Also contains useful information on schools, salary comparisons between cities.
- United States Chamber of Commerce: www.uschamber.org

TOP CITY LIST

List five cities or regions associated with each category.

Proximity to family

_____

_____

_____

_____

_____

Affordability

_____

_____

_____

_____

_____

Weather/climate

_____

_____

_____

_____

_____

Opportunities for
spouse

_____

_____

_____

_____

_____

Quality of schools

_____

_____

_____

_____

_____

Entertainment and
   social opportunities   ————————————

    ————————————

    ————————————

    ————————————

    ————————————

Outdoor activities
   (ski, beach, hike, etc)   ————————————

    ————————————

    ————————————

    ————————————

    ————————————

Airport access   ————————————

    ————————————

    ————————————

    ————————————

    ————————————

Safety/crime   ————————————

    ————————————

    ————————————

    ————————————

    ————————————

Church/synagogue
   mosques   ————————————

    ————————————

    ————————————

    ————————————

    ————————————

Other   _____

           _____

           _____

           _____

           _____

Other   _____

           _____

           _____

           _____

           _____

Other   _____

           _____

           _____

           _____

Your top cities/areas   _____

           _____

           _____

           _____

           _____

           _____

           _____

           _____

           _____

3

WHERE DO YOU WANT TO WORK? FINDING THE IDEAL PRACTICE

Fortunately for job seekers, there are many different types of medical practices to join or start, each with its particular pros and cons. Just as it is important to "know yourself" when finding an ideal practice location, it is crucial to take an inventory of your personality, professional and social goals, and drive when finding the right fit between you and the ideal practice.

There are several types of practice setups. The main categories include the following:

- Solo practitioner (starting your own practice)
- Joining a solo practitioner (single specialty)
- Single specialty, small group practice
- Single specialty, large group practice (often referred to as "mega" groups)
- Multispecialty group practice
- Managed care company employment
- Academic practice
- Locum tenens
- Government (Veterans Affairs, etc.)

SOLO PRACTICE

Starting a solo practice is perhaps one of the most difficult and challenging choices when evaluating career options. It can also be one of the most rewarding, knowing that you have essentially built a practice from scratch. It is also often more demanding, knowing that the responsibility for running, maintaining, and developing the practice begins and ends with you. One of the most important factors for success is identifying the right demographics. You will want to find an area with the type of patients you most want to reach—the elderly, underserved, etc. This information will be available from local hospitals, Chambers of Commerce, and city government. Census information is available on the internet at http://quickfacts.census.gov/. It may also be important to have a financial or banking advisor assist with planning and execution of the business plan. In some instances, solo practice setup may be greatly assisted by Physician Recruitment Agreements, or PRAs, which are discussed later in the text.

Solo practice careers were quite dominant decades ago, but have gradually fallen out of favor over the years as the business, financial, and managed care pressures of running a practice have increased. Starting your own practice involves a significant amount of preparation, and this manual will only serve to point out certain highlights for those individuals. Additional information can also be found from the following groups:

- American Academy of Family Physicians: "On Your Own: Starting a Medical Practice from the Ground Up" at 800-944-0000 or *www.aafp.org/x19744.xml*
- American Medical Association: "Starting a Medical Practice" at 800-621-8335 or *www.amapress.org*
- Medical Economics: "Starting Your Own Practice" at 888-480-0579 or *http://www.memag.com/memag/*

Issues to consider when evaluating a career as a solo practitioner include the time demands on yourself and family while establishing the practice in the first two to 3 years, the need to consider the significant finances and debt incurred during start-up, as well as balancing the need to be both a practitioner as well as a businessperson. For those with the right personality and drive, the path to a solo practice may be quite rewarding.

Pros:

- Pride of being responsible for the growth and development of your own practice.
- Possible financial benefits from running an efficient and streamlined practice.
- Being your own boss.
- Avoidance of interphysician conflicts in running and managing the practice.

Cons:

- Added pressure of being singly responsible for the growth and development of your own practice.
- Maximum efficiency in terms of physician:staff ratio often not achieved in a solo practice—translation: higher costs of practice.
- Responsibility for your own call coverage. Many often set up a loose association with other local practitioners (be aware of local politics and factions that may try to make it difficult for you to establish a practice).
- High start-up costs.
- Financial aspects of setting up your own practice. You (and often, the bank) are responsible for setting up your own practice, which obviously entails a certain degree of financial risk. Alternatively, certain practice start-ups may be assisted by a local hospital physician recruitment agreement (PRA). These agreements pose unique risks and benefits. See the Chapter 9, "Negotiating a Fair and Proper Contract," for more details.
- Potentially several months until revenue stream starts (insurance companies often have 90 days to process claims and make reimbursements).

JOINING A SOLO PRACTICE

Joining a solo practice is a common scenario and affords the benefits of joining a small, single practice, while minimizing some of the headache associated with starting from scratch. This can often be quite beneficial in terms of the efficiencies gained by adding a second partner to a practice, as significant additions to office staff and nursing are often not necessary when adding one additional physician.

When looking at joining a solo practitioner, there are several issues that must be delicately investigated and addressed. First, it is important that the solo practice you are evaluating has a good relationship with both the community that it serves, as well as with the local hospital and physicians. Although it is the exception, solo practitioners may be, on occasion, solo for a reason. It cannot be stressed enough that the job-seeking physician and the solo practitioner see "eye to eye" and can ultimately work together. Personality differences rank near the top when it comes to conflicts in practice management. More than one interview and careful investigation of the local medical environment, including other physicians, local hospitals, and drug company representatives are great sources of information.

Second, it is very important to discuss the future of the practice you are evaluating with the solo practitioner. Although again an exception, there are instances where solo practitioners may try to "dump" a practice on the newcomer, that is, leaving or retiring within a short period. Also investigate any current or impending changes to the dynamic of the practice (lawsuits, billing and collecting issues, government investigation into Medicare/Medicaid practices, etc). It is critical that these are investigated during and after the interview process, as detailed later in the text.

Finally, it is not uncommon for family members to be part of the office or management staff in a solo practice situation. Although the inherent cost-savings are obvious, it is not difficult to see that when a new physician joins a practice, there is potential for preferential treatment (and usually not in your favor). This can range from diverting certain patients to and from your part of the practice, to billing and collection issues, to disciplinary issues. For example, how do you tell your partner's spouse that they come across as rude to patients on the phone? Although a delicate issue, practices with *significant* family involvement should be avoided for the mere potential for conflict. It is not unusual for some well-run practices to have rules against hiring family, even their children, say during summer break.

Pros:

- Established patient and referral base (opportunity to become busy fast)
- Established office and staff (billing, collecting, nursing, etc.)
- Efficiencies of a small group practice (may translate to higher income)
- Help with call coverage
- Benefit of a colleague with whom to consult
- Inherent camaraderie (hopefully)

Cons:

- Often the burden of the new recruit to conform to the norms and operation of the existing practitioner
- Potential personality conflicts
- Potential for preferential call schedule (new recruit may end up with a disproportionate number of weekends or holidays)
- Potential for new recruit to be given a disproportionate number of insurance-poor or problem patients
- Preexisting office or staff politics (beware of family working in the office)

JOINING A SINGLE SPECIALTY, SMALL GROUP PRACTICE

Joining a small, single-specialty practice is often a popular choice among new physicians. It has many of the benefits of a solo practice and often adds value in terms of potential for practice efficiencies, when it is well run. Many practices have a long-term track record and an established reputation (hopefully positive) with the local community, referring physicians, and hospitals.

When they are well run, practice efficiencies in terms of office personnel and nursing can translate to higher long-term income. The caveat to this statement is that there is often a sweet spot in terms of practice efficiency. Under a certain number, employees may be underutilized. Over a certain number, additional employees will need to be hired in order to sustain the workload, thereby increasing certain fixed costs to running a practice. These costs can vary substantially, depending of location (geography) of practice and practice specialty, malpractice, and other costs.

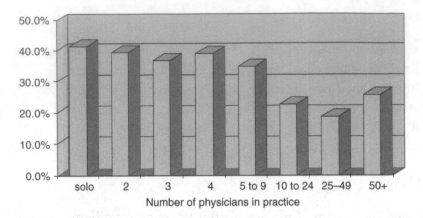

Figure 1   Median Professional Expenses as a Percentage
of Gross.

Figure 1 gives an idea of *average* practice expenses expressed as a percentage of gross, when indexed to the number of physicians in a group. As a rule of thumb, most practices want to keep expenses under 50%; those with significantly higher expenses may raise a red flag.

Pros

• Established reputation and referral patterns
• Established office (personnel, nursing)
• Potential for electronic record keeping and billing
• Resources in terms of advertising, capital investments into practice
• Likelihood of new physician becoming busy fast
• Better ability to negotiate insurance contracts
• Light call schedule
• Flexibility in establishing subspecialty within practice

Cons

• Possibility of conflicts concerning interphysician personality and professional issues

SINGLE SPECIALTY, LARGE GROUP PRACTICE

Joining a mega group, as some may call them, has distinct advantages as well as certain disadvantages. If you're looking to find such a group, they may not exist in certain specialties or geographical areas; in other fields, they are becoming increasingly common. Cardiology, gastroenterology, and large internal medicine groups are common examples. Several factors have driven the formation of these larger groups over the past decade. Cost advantages by sharing overhead and expenses, including fixed costs such as buildings and land, can be significant. In addition, personnel and equipment costs may be maximally utilized, thereby streamlining efficiency. Although subject to various regulations, large groups may be able to negotiate more effectively with insurance carriers in terms of reimbursement rates. This may allow for certain groups to "work smarter, not harder" as reimbursement rates continue to experience continued challenges in the future.

For the newly joining physician, the immediate benefits can include plugging into an established patient and referral base, which can often mean becoming busy in terms of patient load in a short period. Additionally, there may be a certain camaraderie depending on the group dynamic, that allows for consulting with your peers. As the group size increases, there may also be room for physicians to subspecialize within their fields, as different physicians with additional fellowship training or interests become part of the group. Call schedules can often be more favorable in large groups, although the caveat is that the senior most physicians in these groups may often have disproportionately less call time (including holidays and weekends).

Although group size does have many of these benefits, they do come with certain disadvantages, although these may be considered relative depending on your individual practice philosophy, personality, and overall goals. First, as group size increases, the need for additional layers of management increases. This may include nurse managers, practice managers, office managers, separate billing and collection departments, quality control officers, recruiters, and others; all depending on the size and relative sophistication of the group. Some of the tasks may be cross-covered by the physicians in the group; others will require dedicated staff.

The advantage of having such people in the practice, at least in theory, is to physicians to concentrate on patient care. For those who are either averse or otherwise object to the increasing business aspects of medicine, this may be ideal. For those who are more financially savvy, or wish to be more involved in the business and financial workings of their group practice, large groups will often have a formalized structure in which partners can be more involved in this aspect. Regardless of the path you choose, it is *strongly* encouraged that all physicians acquire a basic financial knowledge of the workings of their group and remain involved in the group dynamic. Quite simply, physicians in the modern practice of medicine *cannot* afford to remain insulated as to the financial and business aspects of medicine.

Major downsides of the large group practice stem from the size and additional layers of management that they require. Some individuals may feel that there is a certain lack of group cohesion or closeness; others may feel that their individual ability to change or implement new or different ideas may be limited. These issues vary greatly from practice to practice and are often best investigated by speaking to the junior-most partners within the group. Additional issues may arise from compensation differences between partners and nonpartners, junior and senior partners, and specialists versus nonspecialists. These potential problems may differ based on the compensation formula that a group follows. An example may be reimbursement differences between a fellowship-trained physician who may have a low volume patient load but performs a valuable service to the group and a generalist who may be significantly busier with a larger patient load. These issues are addressed further in the Chapter 9, "Negotiating a Fair and Proper Contract."

Pros:

- Large group size
- Camaraderie, ability to consult others
- Practice efficiency (variable)
- Group insurance reimbursement negotiating ability (variable)

- Established referral base
- Established office setup (billing, collecting, charting, etc.)

Cons:

- Bureaucratic decision-making process (variable)
- Physician compensation issues (variable)

JOINING A MULTISPECIALTY GROUP PRACTICE

As the name suggests, a multispecialty group practice (MSG) is an organization consisting of primary care physicians, surgeons, and specialists, in varying combinations, under one roof. As a result many consultants can often exist together as their own distinct medical community. As with a large group practice, the benefits often include a built-in referral base with an established reputation. Similarly, a large MSG will often have leverage in terms of insurance reimbursement rates, as well as inherent cost savings in certain areas. Some may also have additional revenue streams from lab, radiology, and other facilities. Established methods of billing, collecting, and charting are also common. As group size and sophistication increases, other benefits such as disability plans, health insurance, and various retirement plans may also be available.

An MSG typically also has a formal governance structure. This may be a benefit for those physicians wishing to be less involved in the business aspect of medicine and more focused on their practice. For those wishing to be more involved in the business area, there are frequently opportunities to be active in the governance of the group. Regardless of the path chosen, it is strongly encouraged for the physician to remain aware and involved in the financial aspects of the practice.

For specialists who depend on a steady stream of referrals, a general rule of thumb is that approximately 50% of the group should be devoted to primary care. As community referrals into the MSG may be minimal, the internal referral pattern of the group should be able to support specialist volume. Specialists will also often serve to balance the higher overhead of primary physicians.

Management of MSGs can vary. Two main types exist: those owned and managed by physicians, and those controlled by a physician management company. As the latter tend to have a more volatile relationship and history, it is important to investigate the history and future plans for MSGs run by management corporations.

Finally, physician compensation issues may be variable depending on the MSG. Large groups often have greater bargaining power with managed care plans, ability to reinvest income in medical equipment, medical systems, and quality improvement. The tradeoff is that overhead costs can be somewhat greater, depending on the management structure and operational style of a particular MSG. Specialists may sometimes find their compensation somewhat less than those of their peers in a community. Negotiating a fair and appropriate contract is important in these situations and is outlined separately in Chapter 9, "Negotiating a Fair and Proper Contract."

Pros:

- Large group size
- Ability to consult within group
- Group insurance reimbursement negotiating ability
- Established referral base
- Established office setup (billing, collecting, charting, etc.)

Cons:

- Bureaucratic decision-making process
- Physician compensation issues
- Lack of participation in profit from ancillary services such as dialysis centers, radiology facilities, lithotripters, etc.

ACADEMIC PRACTICE

Academic appointments can take several different forms including full-time or part-time positions, as well as clinical versus consultative appointments. These are specialty-dependent and can vary tremendously depending on the particular academic center. Most traditional faculty positions are tenure-tracked and include research opportunities, clinical obligations, teaching, and administrative responsibilities in some combination, depending on the needs and goals of the department.

The pathways of the tenure track can vary depending on the institution and specific department involved. These traditional academic appointments usually begin with an eventual goal to achieve the status of professor of the given specialty. Most positions usually start at the rank of assistant professor directly out of residency. This is the lowest seniority rank of the tenure track. In order to advance appropriately, you must submit an application, typically referred to as a *dossier* to an advancement or promotions committee, which votes on and recommends promotion. In the dossier, you submit all of the achievements and performance data as an assistant professor and request advancement to the next higher rank of associate professor. The promotions committee reviews the data and determines whether you have accomplished sufficient achievement to merit advancement. Advancement criteria may include research or other publications, amount of research grants and funding, fulfilling teaching obligations, clinical productivity, charitable activity, administrative responsibility either locally, within the institution, or nationally. Most successful applicants typically demonstrate achievements in multiple categories. Individuals typically spend between three and 7 years as an assistant professor before successful advancement to associate professor. Beware that advancement is not guaranteed and you may be required to submit applications to the promotions committee multiple times before advancing.

The position of associate professor typically involves slightly more administrative responsibility but does vary tremendously between institutions. Individuals may spend between five to 20 plus years in this position before advancing to full professor status. This next advancement process is similar in steps to that previously described to advance from assistant professor to associate professor. However, the advancement to full professor is far more stringent and difficult, requiring many more achievements and accomplishments especially in the research arena and in participation with national specialty societies. Again, there is no guarantee for advancement.

The ranking and track record of successful tenure of the faculty may be an important piece of information for you as an applicant. Since the promotion process of the tenure track can be quite variable between institutions, it behooves you to investigate the criteria and process for academic advancement within a particular institution before proceeding. Specifically, you should seek to identify the institutional and departmental biases toward research, publications, grants, community service, and clinical productivity, and determine if those goals are comparable with your goals. If they are congruent, there is a higher probability of promotion and thus you should consider the position. If not, then perhaps you should investigate a position at another institution.

Academic positions can be salaried or incentive-structured based on productivity. It is important to know that many opportunities can be created, depending on your and the institution's particular needs and interests. Academic practices definitely pay less than private practice; however, there are other benefits that may provide nonmonetary utility. For example, academic practices typically provide the opportunity to teach and perform research. Additionally, residents and students, as well as ancillary support staff, are present to help with "busy" work. With that said, it is important to understand that with controlled resident work hours and decreases in reimbursement, the amount of support staff has been dwindling and can vary tremendously from institution to institution. Nowadays, much of the academic lifestyle has changed and more resembles private practice in terms of emphasis on clinical work and productivity.

Another nonmonetary benefit found in most academic practices is the mentoring of young staff. Since most academic practices tend to be group structured with multiple, different faculty of varying experience, interests, and goals, a fertile advanced training and mentoring environment exists for a young physician. This can be beneficial for a young practitioner as it fosters an advanced learning opportunity with independence tempered with guidance and support.

Also, since most academic practices are large group practices with multiple physicians, residents, and fellows, the burden of call coverage may be lessened. Typically, the call may be split with more physicians thus reducing the frequency of on-call days. In addition, the presence of residents or fellows may serve as primary "buffers" from the burden of direct emergency room and phone coverage responsibilities. Again, a prospective individual should investigate the varying talents of the faculty and inquire about the on-call structure, frequency, and severity.

Important points to evaluate in an academic practice include clinical volume, political structure, leadership stability, and research opportunities. In terms of the training program itself, look at the quality of the residents, the overall program, structure, and stability. Have an understanding of the institution, as well as the leaderships' attitude and expectations of the faculty.

Pros:

- Student, resident interaction and teaching
- Decreased need to manage the financial aspect of medicine, compared to private practice
- Stable compensation
- Possibility of decreased call responsibilities
- Potential better benefits such as retirement, health insurance, etc.
- Increased complexity and intellectual challenge of cases in academia
- Advanced learning opportunity with independence, balanced with an environment of guidance and support

Cons:

- Increasing need to meet revenue targets while maintaining research, teaching, and administrative duties
- Usually, no chance for partnership
- Often billing/collecting ratios are substandard in academia, compared to private practice
- Challenging road to tenure
- Political structure and issues
- Restrictive covenants, if present, may be broad
- Possibility of decreased salary when compared to private sector

LOCUM TENENS (FLEXIBLE CONTRACTS INVOLVING VARYING DURATION AND GEOGRAPHY)

Pros:

- Freedom of work location and schedule
- Freedom from administrative, financial, and other headaches
- Liability, malpractice usually covered
- Housing, car, and other expenses often covered

Cons:

- Need to be flexible in terms of different work environments
- Limited opportunity to develop long-term relationships with patients and colleagues
- Usually limited health and other long-term benefits
- May be difficult to arrange when considering spouse, children, and other needs

GOVERNMENT (VETERANS AFFAIRS, PUBLIC SERVICE, ETC.)

Pros:

- Potential academic affiliation, providing for stimulating teaching duties
- Generous benefit packages
- Stable salary
- Decreased need to hit production, financial targets
- Sense of civic duty
- Stable hours and work schedule
- Possibility of student loan/educational debt forgiveness

Cons:

- Stable salary
- Possibility of decreased autonomy, and need to function according to strict protocols and guidelines
- Position may take on a certain monotony over time

4
THE CURRICULUM VITAE

It's important to prepare a well-written resume or curriculum vitae (CV) prior to applying for a position. For the majority of young physicians and residents, a one or two page resume detailing education, work experience, and licensure is sufficient. However, if you are an established physician, or if you have been involved in extensive research, presentations, and have other skill-sets, prepare a formal CV. A CV includes the basics of a resume, but detailed experiences will add several additional pages of information.

The first thing to prepare is a cover letter (see Fig. 1). This letter should emphasize your accomplishments without appearing overly grandiose or self-centered. A good way to achieve this is to show how the group's needs interface with your particular interests and strengths. For example, "Your group's need for a specialist in oncology fits well with my experience and fellowship training in this field." Cover letters should be limited to a single page and should include your e-mail address and office/contact numbers. The letter should be signed in black ink.

Understand that the cover letter serves as a lead-in for the CV, which will provide details about your qualifications. Many physicians tend to provide too much information or fail to prioritize it appropriately. You don't want someone to leaf through several pages of information before finding the facts that are most relevant to the position to which you are applying.

Your CV should be tailored to the type of position you are seeking. For example, if you are interested in an academic position, you should emphasize your teaching and research experiences (see Fig. 2). If you are seeking a private practice position, listing your ambulatory care experience as well as procedural experience may be more important (see Fig. 3).

In general, a CV should start by listing demographic information, including contact addresses and numbers, followed by education with degrees, and outline of postgraduate training, and relevant certifications or board eligibility. Following this, the content of a CV will vary depending on the career track you are pursuing. Examples of sections to potentially add to a CV include *Practice Experience*, listing ambulatory sites and preceptors; *Procedural Skills*, listing procedures credentialed by your program, as well as procedures you are competent in; *Administrative Positions*, listing committees on which you have served, supervisory roles, and projects in which you have been involved; and *Teaching Experience*, listing conferences, research interests, abstracts, papers, chapters, etc. that you have contributed to or written.

It is important to keep your CV looking professional. Pay attention to small details, including spelling and punctuation. Use consistent fonts and headings. Use a laser printer instead of an inkjet, which can smear. Last, spend a little extra on high quality bond white, or light-colored, paper.

It's also helpful to keep your CV relevant, updating it periodically with your accomplishments, lectures, articles, etc.

Once your interview is finished, it is always recommended to send a thank you letter, even if you are not interested. Understand that medicine is a small world, and you may end up practicing in the same community or area, not to mention seeing these same people at professional meetings. Keeping up a good reputation and image with your colleagues is good practice.

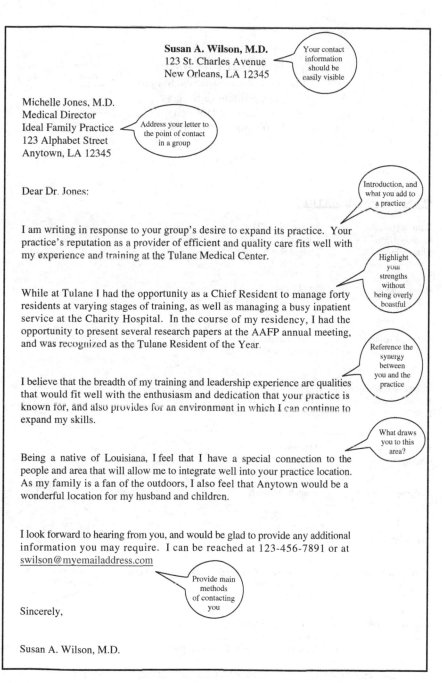

Susan A. Wilson, M.D.
123 St. Charles Avenue
New Orleans, LA 12345

Your contact information should be easily visible

Michelle Jones, M.D.
Medical Director
Ideal Family Practice
123 Alphabet Street
Anytown, LA 12345

Address your letter to the point of contact in a group

Dear Dr. Jones:

Introduction, and what you add to a practice

I am writing in response to your group's desire to expand its practice. Your practice's reputation as a provider of efficient and quality care fits well with my experience and training at the Tulane Medical Center.

Highlight your strengths without being overly boastful

While at Tulane I had the opportunity as a Chief Resident to manage forty residents at varying stages of training, as well as managing a busy inpatient service at the Charity Hospital. In the course of my residency, I had the opportunity to present several research papers at the AAFP annual meeting, and was recognized as the Tulane Resident of the Year.

Reference the synergy between you and the practice

I believe that the breadth of my training and leadership experience are qualities that would fit well with the enthusiasm and dedication that your practice is known for, and also provides for an environment in which I can continue to expand my skills.

What draws you to this area?

Being a native of Louisiana, I feel that I have a special connection to the people and area that will allow me to integrate well into your practice location. As my family is a fan of the outdoors, I also feel that Anytown would be a wonderful location for my husband and children.

I look forward to hearing from you, and would be glad to provide any additional information you may require. I can be reached at 123-456-7891 or at swilson@myemailaddress.com

Provide main methods of contacting you

Sincerely,

Susan A. Wilson, M.D.

Figure 1   Sample Cover Letter.

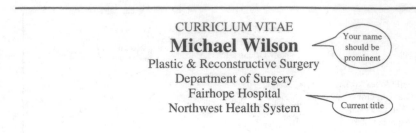

CURRICLUM VITAE
Michael Wilson
Plastic & Reconstructive Surgery
Department of Surgery
Fairhope Hospital
Northwest Health System

Your name should be prominent

Current title

PERSONAL INFORMATION

Date of Birth:	March 21, 1971
Place of Birth:	Cleveland, Ohio
Citizenship:	United States

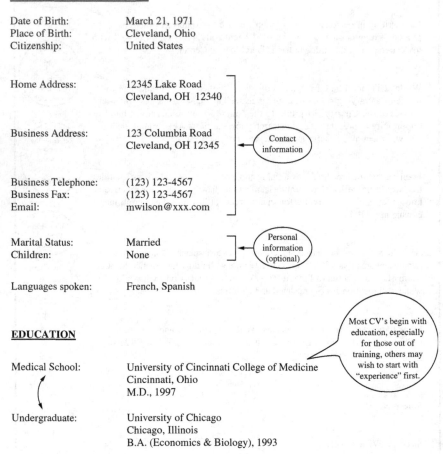

Home Address:	12345 Lake Road Cleveland, OH 12340
Business Address:	123 Columbia Road Cleveland, OH 12345
Business Telephone:	(123) 123-4567
Business Fax:	(123) 123-4567
Email:	mwilson@xxx.com

Contact information

Marital Status:	Married
Children:	None

Personal information (optional)

Languages spoken:	French, Spanish

EDUCATION

Most CV's begin with education, especially for those out of training, others may wish to start with "experience" first.

Medical School:	University of Cincinnati College of Medicine Cincinnati, Ohio M.D., 1997
Undergraduate:	University of Chicago Chicago, Illinois B.A. (Economics & Biology), 1993

Figure 2   Sample CV for Academic Applications (*Continued*).

POST GRADUATE TRAINING

Start with your most recent training and work backwards

Internship: General Surgery
                       Fairhope Hospital, Ohio Clinic Health System
                       Department of Surgery
                       Cleveland, Ohio
                       PGY-1 (1997–1998)

Residency: General Surgery Residency

                       Plastic & Reconstructive Surgery Residency
                       University of Colorado Health Sciences Center
                       Division of Plastic & Reconstructive Surgery
                       Denver, Colorado
                       PGY-4 (2000–2001)
                       PGY-5 Administrative Chief Resident (2001–2002)

                       Fairhope Hospital, Cleveland Clinic Health System
                       Department of Surgery
                       Cleveland, Ohio
                       PGY-2 (1998–1999)
                       PGY-3 (1999–2000)

Additional Training: Aesthetic Surgery Rotation (1999)
                       Ohio Clinic for Aesthetic and Plastic Surgery
                       Westlake, Ohio
                       Preceptor: Joe Davis, M.D.

                       AO ASIF Maxillofacial Course on Treatment of Maxillofacial Trauma &
                       Reconstruction, Chicago, Illinois
                       (July, 2001)

HONORS AND AWARDS

List, with most recent, working backwards

1996   Honorable Mention, for Top Medical Student Cost Effective Medicine
              Research Paper Competition, University of Cincinnati College of Medicine.
              "Effective and Appropriate Use of Antibiotics Utilizing Evidence-Based Medicine"

1994   Fairhope General Hospital Investigational Research Grant. "The Risk of Breast
              Cancer Based on Physical Examination and Mammography: A Retrospective
              Analysis."

1992–1993   Dean's List
              University of Chicago

PROFESSIONAL LICENSURE

State of Ohio, License Number xxx-xxx, Active Status (First Issued 1998)
State of Colorado, License Number xxx-xxx, Active Status (First Issued 2000)

PROFESSIONAL CERTIFICATION

2004   Board Eligible for Certification by American Board of Plastic Surgery
2004   Completion of American Board of Plastic Surgery Written Exam
1998   Completion of USMLE Steps 1, 2 and 3

Figure 2   *(Continued)*

ACADEMIC APPOINTMENTS

2004–current   Clinical Faculty, General Surgery Residency Program
Fairview Hospital Department of Surgery
Ohio Clinic Health System
Cleveland, Ohio

> Important for those considering academia

2002–2004   Assistant Professor of Plastic & Reconstructive Surgery
University of Northwest Health Sciences Center
Denver, Colorado

2003–2004   Clinical Practice Director, Plastic & Reconstructive Surgery
University of Northwest Health Sciences Center
Denver, Colorado

HOSPITAL APPOINTMENTS

2004–current   Attending Surgeon, Plastic & Reconstructive Surgery
Fairhope Hospital, Ohio Clinic Health System, Cleveland, OH
Lakefair Hospital, Ohio Clinic Health System, Cleveland, OH

2002–2004   Attending Surgeon, Plastic & Reconstructive Surgery
University Hospital – Northwest Health Sciences Center, Denver, CO

OTHER APPOINTMENTS

2004-current   Lake View Academy Advisory Council

2004   Northwest College of Medicine Surgical Society
Guest Speaker, "A career in Plastic & Reconstructive Surgery:
Applied Art and Anatomy".
March 1, 2004

HOSPITAL COMMITTEES

2002–current   University Hospital—Pharmacy and Therapeutics Advisory Panel

Figure 2   *(Continued)*

MEMBERSHIP IN SOCIETIES

American Society of Plastic Surgeons (Candidate)
American Society of Aesthetic Plastic Surgeons (Candidate)
Ohio Plastic Surgery Society (Candidate)

PUBLICATIONS

The following subsections can be added as appropriate, more so for those pursuing academics

1.   Wilson, M., Jones, R. "Delayed bleeding following
       laparoscopic cholecystectomy. Abstract published in *Surgical Endoscopy* 1999; 12: 678.

TEXTBOOK CHAPTERS

List most recent, first

2.   Wilson, M, Gordon RV: Upper Extremity Amputation. In *Vascular Hand Surgery* 6th Edition,
       Rutherford MS (editor), Elsevier, Inc. Philadelphia, PA. Chapter 174, 2004.

PRESENTATIONS

1.   Wilson, M, Miller, J. "The Risk of Breast Cancer: A retrospective Analysis."
       A poster presentation at the Annual Breast Cancer Symposium, Houston, Texas,
       December 11–14, 1999.

PHILANTHROPY PROJECTS

1999   Surgical Volunteer Mission to El Complito, Mexico
              TIGA International

REFERENCES

          Larry Jones, M.D.
          Northwest Health Sciences Center
          Chief, Section of Plastic & Reconstructive Surgery
          12345 Main Street
          Denver, Colorado 12345
          (123)456-7890

You will need three reliable references

Figure 2   *(Continued)*

Curriculum Vitae

Michael Wilson, M.D.

Name easily visible

BIOGRAPHICAL DATA:
Date of Birth: 6/6/1970
Marital Status: Single

Optional

HOME ADDRESS & TELEPHONE:
12340 Alameda
Houston, Texas 70000
(555) 123-4567

Contact info easily visible

ACADEMIC APPOINTMENTS:

SOUTHERN UNIVERSITY SCHOOL OF MEDICINE – DEPT. OF NEUROLOGY, New Orleans, LA
Clinical Instructor

CLINICAL APPOINTMENTS:

Listing, from most recent, working backwards

NORTH TEXAS MEDICAL CENTER, Houston, TX
Chief of Service, Department of Neurology

POSTGRADUATE EDUCATION:

SOUTHERN UNIVERSITY SCHOOL OF MEDICINE – DEPT. OF NEUROLOGY, New Orleans, LA
Neurology residency, July 2000–June 2004

SOUTHERN UNIVERSITY SCHOOL OF MEDICINE – DEPT. OF GENERAL SURGERY, New Orleans, LA
General Surgery resident, July 1998–June 2000

GRADUATE EDUCATION:

BOSTON UNIVERSITY SCHOOL OF MEDICINE, Boston, MA
Degree - Doctor of Medicine, May 1998

UNDERGRADUATE EDUCATION:

BOSTON UNIVERSITY, Boston, MA
Bachelor of Science in Human Physiology, May 1994

List all pertinent achievements

HONORS:
International Volunteers in Neurology, Traveling Fellowship Recipient, 2004
Nominated for Humanitarianism in Teaching Award, Southern School of Medicine, 2004
Neurological Medicine Society of North America - 2003 Inaugural Traveling Fellowship Recipient
Society for Neurological Studies -2001 Inaugural Traveling Fellowship Recipient

Figure 3 Sample CV for Private Practice Applications.

PUBLICATION AND LECTURE EXPERIENCE:

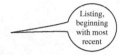
Listing, beginning with most recent

DEPARTMENT OF NEUROLOGY – November 2004
Southern University School of Medicine, New Orleans, LA
  Presentation: *Neurologic Outcomes and Analysis after Acute Hemiparesis*
  Mendez, F., **Wilson, M.,** Thomas, R.
  Status: Presented at 2004 22nd World Congress on Neurology

DEPARTMENT OF NEUROLOGY – May 2004
Southern University School of Medicine, New Orleans, LA
  Moderated Poster Presentation: *"Advances in Parkinson's Disease Management"*
  Wilson, M.., Morey, A., Jones, L., Hellstrom, W.
  Status: Presented at 2004 National ANA annual meeting.

DEPARTMENT OF NEUROLOGY – April 2001
Southern University School of Medicine, New Orleans, LA
  Abstract: *"Use of Aspirin to Reduce Risk of CVA."*
  Davis, R., **Wilson, M.,** Thomas, R.
  Status: Presented at 2001 Southeastern Section ANA annual meeting.

List all pertinent, start with most recent

APPOINTMENTS:

AMERICAN ASSOCIATION OF NEUROLOGISTS   2004–05

Young Physician Section Convention Chairperson

LOUISIANA EDUCATION EARLY DETECTION AND RESEARCH MTG   2003

Guest Lecturer

GRADUATE MEDICAL EDUCATION COMMITTEE   2003–04
Resident Liason Member

SOUTHERN MEDICAL CENTER PHARMACEUTICAL AND THERAPEUTICS   2002–03
COMMITTEE
Resident Liason Member

BOSTON UNIVERSITY PRE-MEDICAL SOCIETY
President   1992–93
Vice President   1991–92

CERTIFICATIONS/LICENSURE

List all pertinent

Certified by the American Board of Neurology   2005
Licensed by the State of Louisiana   2002
Licensed by the State of Texas   2001
USMLE, Part I, II, III   1997–99

MEMBERSHIPS

American Neurological Association
Neurologic Society of North America

Figure 3   *(Continued)*.

5
STARTING YOUR SEARCH

As mentioned in the timeline in Chapter 1, it is important to have time on your side with the job search. Although conventional wisdom says that more time is better than less, too often even candidates with well planned searches can find themselves short of time. Common scenarios include having a contract fall through at the last minute, or involve a change in personal or professional circumstances. Having irreconcilable differences arise when it comes to contract negotiations and subsequently being left with no alternatives late in the game is a situation to avoid. The best advice for those starting the search is to do so *at least 1 year or greater in advance*. When it comes to starting the search, understand that it does not imply that you need to start interviewing that far ahead; indeed, it implies that you need to start asking questions, making initial contacts, and taking a personal inventory of your particular career needs.

LOCATING LEADS

When it comes to asking questions, who do you turn to for leads? Well, as it often turns out, some of your best sources are right around you. This includes graduating or graduated residents who have recently "gone out there" ahead of you. They will often be the best gauges of the current market, including "hot" areas, and perhaps most importantly, areas or groups to avoid. They are a good source of current and fair salary ranges to expect as well. Many physicians will often have had multiple offers, with several being quite good, but for whatever reason, not quite right.

They, in effect, may have done much of the legwork for you already, by putting you in touch with some of these groups.

Another excellent source of information can come from the staff physicians with whom you work at your various rotations. They will often have a network of physicians both locally as well as nationally. In addition, they may know people in the government, academic, and private sectors who can prove to be valuable contacts. As most physicians in the modern age of medicine often change careers at various times, they can also serve as a candid source of comparison between the different sectors of practice. As it is human nature to be opinionated, it is important that you speak to as many people as possible before forming any decisions of your own.

Another excellent source of information, but often overlooked, are the pharmaceutical, or industry representatives that most of us come into contact with on a routine basis. These individuals often spend good portions of their day calling on physicians in many different practice situations. As such, they will often be able to provide a reasonable idea of which practices run more efficiently than others, which ones remain busy, etc. As always, it is best to temper advice by speaking to as many individuals as possible. If you are looking into a different geographical area than the one you are currently in, a pharmaceutical representative can always contact their peers in another area. Another benefit of speaking to these individuals is that, although subject to bias, they can provide a relatively independent idea as to the particular dynamic of a certain group or individual.

You will often find that some of the best positions available are not widely advertised or well known. In fact, many groups may be thinking of hiring in the near future, but have not actively recruited as of yet. This is a perfect example of creating your own opportunity and taking a proactive approach to your career search. An excellent way to accomplish this is to draft a letter of introduction and interest to those groups that you may be interested in within a particular city or geographic region. You may want to include your curriculum vitae (CV) with the letter, or provide it upon request. If you are unsure of which groups are in particular area, great sources are your specialty association, the local yellow pages, and of course, the Internet .

RECRUITERS

Recruiters are often a major source of referrals for physicians. Interestingly enough, it usually will not be necessary to find them, as they will often have a way of finding you. The major benefit of utilizing a recruiter for your search is that a good one will often do a lot of the leg work for you. Whether you use one recruiter, or several, is up to you, as they may each have access to different opportunities. Just be aware of the bother factor of having to juggle multiple phone calls, e-mails, letters, and frankly pestering that you may have to deal with on occasion. It is not unusual to have several agents from the *same company* call you several times a week. Regardless, it is advisable to limit yourself to two to three recruiters. Last, *never sign an exclusive agreement with a recruiter.*

So, how do you go about picking the ideal recruiter? It's difficult to decide just based upon fancy mailings or ads, but there are several questions that are prudent to ask:

1. **How long has your group been in business?**   Experience is key, and at least 5 years of industry experience is important. It is also important to ask how long the particular recruiter has been in the industry, and with the particular company. Asking how many physicians the firm and or recruiter places each year is also important.
2. **Who pays for the services?**   Although rare, it is ill-advised to work with a recruiter who charges you. Instead, the fees usually come from the employer.
3. **How long do recruited physicians stay with practices you place them with?**   Obviously, short-term placements are a red-flag that the process used is flawed. Prudent recruiters should spend time investigating your needs and the particular practice to ensure a good fit. Avoid recruiters who persistently "slam" you with offers that have little to do with your individual needs.

4. **How much do you know about the recruiting practice?** You would be surprised by the number of recruiters who do little home-work on the practice opportunities they present you with. Without sounding too pessimistic, it is important that either you or the recruiter delve into the history of a practice. How did the opportunity in the group arise? Is there a significant history of turnover? Are there group dynamic and personality issues? Financial issues?

   If you leave it to the recruiter to find these answers for you, the answers they receive are often taken face value from the head of the medical practice. Answers such as "The previous doctor left because his or her spouse didn't like the area" are common, and can often hide a more complicated truth. If the recruiter doesn't find out, you need to find these answers and more, on your own. No one will "watch your back" like you do.

5. **What is your experience with my specialty or geographic area?** Professional recruiting firms will often have dedicated individuals in a certain field or area.

6. **What is your policy on distributing CVs?** Recruiters may often disseminate CVs indiscriminately. This is especially easy with the Internet. Your CV could easily become distributed widely to various Web sites and communities without your knowledge. As personally identifiable information is often present, it could only compound your problems with other recruiters "circling the prey." Ensure that your CV is sent out only with your permission.

7. **How often can I expect to hear from you?** This can vary from min-imal contact, to something that borders on harassment. It is not unusual to receive multiple phone calls each day from various recruiters, all the way to being paged in the hospital, sometimes under false pretenses. Obviously finding a reasonable balance is important. Unless urgent, it is probably prudent not to readily dis-tribute pager or work numbers to recruiters.

Once you specify certain qualifications such as geography, salary, and group type, the recruiter can often search databases, as well as cold-calling, to provide you with a list of opportunities.

PITFALLS

It is important to remember that when dealing with recruiters, even under the best of intentions, their goal is to put you into a job. Unfortunately, this may not always be the *right* job. With the knowledge that most commissions range from *20 to 30%* of the physicians' salary, it is not difficult to do the math and figure that there is tremendous drive to get you placed. Even in the best of hands, it is critical that you do your own background work prior to signing with a group.

6

PREPARING FOR THE INTERVIEW

Getting to the interview stage is a great milestone in the search process. It is enjoyable in terms of travel and meeting new people, but it also entails a fair amount of work. You will want to obtain more than one interview prior to deciding which position is the best. As most candidates will not have a reference point as to the ideal practice as of yet, multiple interviews will give you the best chance to compare and contrast various opportunities.

The interview process should really be called an *evaluation process*, where the practice evaluates you, and vice versa. It can be broken down into *four components*. The *first* involves you, and the impression you give to the group—a general feeling that comes out over the course of the interview. This requires a bit of advance preparation on your part. You should be prepared to articulate your strengths and weaknesses, including what you wish to add to the group. It is advisable that you arrive to the interview with time to spare and have an attaché or folio with a notepad to take notes. Having additional CVs for the group is also advised.

An important point to know is that if you have gotten to the interview stage with a group, it is likely that they have been favorably impressed by your CV (refer to Chapter 4 for details on creating an appropriate medical curriculum vitae). At this point, the interview serves not only to reinforce the highlights of your achievement as a *physician*, but perhaps more importantly, to validate you as an *individual* with whom they would enjoy working with on a daily basis. As personality conflicts rank high in terms of discord within a group, it is easy to see that a major point of the interview is to see if you are some-one they can work with. Apart from the intangible factor of being a good "fit," being articulate, well dressed, and well mannered all come out in the course of the interview. Just as you have a lot on the line, the group wants to make sure you will be a good steward of their patients and reputation.

In summary, organizations want a candidate who:

- Is trained well.
- Will be liked by their patients.
- Gets along with their peers, faculty, etc.
- Enjoys the practice of medicine.
- Has a strong work ethic.
- Works well in a group setting.
- If married, has a spouse who also desires to be in that area.
- Has his or her own reasons or desires to move to that area.

INTERVIEW QUESTIONS

Typical questions you may want to rehearse prior to the interview (and what the interviewer may be trying to extract from the question):

- So, tell me about yourself?
  - o   Basic and common opening question.
  - o   Attempt to get to know you, your personality, and your people skills.
- Where are you from?
  - o   Do you have anything in common with the group?
  - o   What type of environment did you grow up in?
  - o   Is it nearby this opportunity?
- What are your strengths?
  - o   Give examples, clinical or otherwise, where you excel.
- What are your weaknesses?
  - o   Honest, but simple examples.
  - o   Be prepared to discuss ways you have worked or are working to overcome them.

- Why do you want to join this practice?
  - o General idea to see if you've thought the decision through—have you really done your homework and is Timbuktu someplace you really would like to be?
- What draws you to this particular area of the country?
  - o Again, to see if there is a legitimate reason for your interviewing (you didn't interview in Hawaii just for the free trip...it really happens).
- Why do you want to change jobs (if appropriate)?
  - o Any skeletons in the closet?
- What are your clinical interests and proficiencies?
  - o What do you bring to the group?
- What does your family think of you practicing in this location?
  - o Will you stay here, or will there be family pressure to move?
- What are you looking for in a practice?
  - o Another general question to gauge your state of preparedness.
  - o How would you fit in here?
  - o What are your expectations?

For those pursuing a career in academia, additional questions to consider:

- What are your research goals and aims?
- What sources of funding are you anticipating?
- What teaching experience do you have, and what teaching qualities do you possess?
- Where do you find yourself in the next 5 to 10 years?

PREPARING ANSWERS

Now that the group has had a chance to find out about you, let's move on to the *second* portion of the process. This is where you really need to do your homework ahead of the interview. Use the Internet, medical colleagues, pharmaceutical representatives, nursing staff—just about anybody who has had contact with some facet of the group—as a guide.

Some questions are common and expected early in the interview process. Other questions are more detailed and probing, and it is understandable if partners hesitate to discuss them with you immediately. Gauge the situation, and proceed accordingly. Some in-depth financial and reimbursement questions may best be answered during a follow-up visit if both you and the group express continued interest.

Typical questions to consider asking include the following:

- What qualities are you looking for in a new partner?
- You currently have X partners. When was the last time you added someone to your group and why? How many physicians have left in the last 3 to 5 years?
  - o These are some of the most important questions to ask, in terms of determining the stability of a group. A pattern of frequent turnover by either medical staff or physicians is a red flag. Being able to speak to recently exited physicians is priceless. It is not unheard of for groups to hire an employee and make certain promises, including eventual partnership. Later, they may find it more financially beneficial to terminate the contract rather than offer partnership, and instead, hire another employee. Some groups may not even intend (covertly) to offer partnership to employees. Although not exact, a sign of this may manifest itself in employee turnover that occurs every 2 to 5 years.
- What is the community need for physicians in my specialty?
  - o You will need to be able to gauge the competitive environment of the practice. What is the group's share of the market? Who are the other major players in the area?
- What is your relationship with other similar groups in town?
  - o Look for nonconfrontational, collegial responses; hostility may indicate problems.
- I noticed you have multiple sites. Do you all practice at multiple locations, or are you assigned a location?
  - o Typical problem encountered *after* signing on: Guess which doctor gets to be the new "gopher" in the group? Know *before* you sign!

- How many hospitals does the group serve?
  - o What is the quality of the medical, nursing, and administration at each hospital? How are the hospitals doing financially? Have there, or will there be, mergers? You will want to make sure that the group is well positioned in viable, progressive, and well-run facilities.
- How is the call and vacation schedule organized?
  - o Delicate question, but it needs to be tactfully posed at some point. It is not unusual for senior most partners to "back off" call a bit, sometimes not taking weekends or certain holidays. Again, know *before* you sign.
- Is there a certain patient load that I will be expected to handle?
  - o Phrase this tactfully, as not to appear lazy (unless you are).
  - o Seriously speaking, this may come into play in groups that have a large "capitated" practice. In this case, patient volume plays a more significant role.
- Will all my patients be new referrals, or will I take on established patients from the group?
  - o Again here is another delicate point and one that is hard to ask. It is not unusual for the new physician to assume patients that are problematic, new patients with lower reimbursement insurance, a larger percentage of Medicare, Medicaid, or no insurance at all. Your best defense is joining a group that appears to have a high ethical and moral standard. That means trusting your sixth sense.
- What percentage of the practice's payers are managed care, fee-for-service, Medicare, and Medicaid?
  - o This will vary depending on your specialty and geography; look out for practices that fall significantly outside the norm (unless, of course you are looking for a group with those patient populations).
- What is the managed care environment, or penetration?
  - o Have health plans driven down reimbursements in this community and caused physicians to leave (maybe causing the vacancy you're taking).
- What is your current overhead rate, and are the partners satisfied with that?

- o   Remember, rates over 50% are generally excessive, and the lower, the better.
- Are partners satisfied with their incomes?
  - o   A general open-ended question to gain a group philosophy—are they primarily money-driven (watch out), or does no one really care (watch out)?
- How long have the doctors and clinical and administrative personnel been with the practice?
  - o   Perhaps one of the most important questions: it is critical to read between the lines here. Look out for answers that appear to "dodge the ball," or otherwise give flimsy answers. Typically shady answers leave it at a brief, "His or her spouse didn't like it here," etc. A huge red flag is a group who has had several physicians recently enter and leave the group. There is also a strong correlation between how well the group is run and staff (nursing, office personnel) turnover. Abusive physician staff, low morale, and other problems can manifest themselves in turnover.
- Have any of the senior partners announced retirement plans? If so, what is their timetable for retirement.
  - o   Although planned retirement is inevitable, just make sure that your arriving doesn't coincide with a senior partner's "golden parachute," or quick escape plan. Yes, that happens too. You also need to ask (covered in Chapter 8) what the buy-out for that senior physician is (you may be helping to pay for his or her retirement).
- Does the practice plan to expand, and could I play a part of that?
  - o   And how much will it cost me to play? It would be good to know ahead of time if all the physicians in a group are expected to put in thousands of dollars into a new dialysis center, surgical center, or new equipment, for example. Senior physicians may have saved up a significant amount of money over the years, but major outlays of cash may impact a new physician considerably more.
- Is the group involved in other joint ventures or ancillary services?
  - o   For various reasons, these are becoming more common, and include lab, radiology, ambulatory surgical centers, and a variety of other ventures. This can be a complicated area, mainly in a

legal and regulatory sense. Make sure this portion of a contract is carefully looked over by you and a contract attorney.

o   In most instances, you will not be sharing in the revenue from these sources until you become a partner. Clarify.

- What is the timetable and formula for buying into the practice?
   o   *Critical!* Refer to Chapter 9, "Negotiating a Fair and Proper Contract" and research *thoroughly* prior to signing.
- How are income and expenses divided among physicians?
   o   Some groups divide expenses based on productivity (indirectly tying expenses to resource utilization—nurses, supplies, etc.) while others split expenses evenly. The only problem with the latter is that not all physicians are similar, and thereby they work and utilize resources differently. Something to consider.
- What is the benefits package?
   o   This can be quite simple or complex, depending on the situation. We'll look into this in detail in Chapter 9.

Note that questions regarding compensation come last. Otherwise, you may come across as somewhat aggressive and concerned only with the bottom line. It is significantly more important to learn about the practice and its patients and to determine if this is a place you would want to work. Unless there is truly something wrong with the practice, the money will come; you just don't want to find yourself significantly outside the norm.

If you get some one-on-one time with a doctor, you might ask, "What do you like best about working here?" Or "What bothers you most about this job?" Believe it or not, it is quite informative and revealing to ask the office staff the same questions if you get a stolen moment.

For those pursuing a career in academia, additional questions to consider:

- What is the success rate for academic promotion within the department or division?
- What are the criteria for promotion with the department or division?
- What are the teaching and research obligations?

- How does the faculty incentive plan work?
- What is the system of taxation within the institution, and how much are the various taxes?
- What opportunities for "hard funding" or salary support are available within the institution or department?
- What are the opportunities for leadership at the institution (if desired)?
- What are the provisions for support if residents are not available due to work hour restrictions? Are there physician assistants or nurse practitioners available to distribute some of the clinical burden?

WORK SURROUNDINGS

So now that the group has had a chance to investigate you thoroughly and, hopefully, you've had a chance to turn the tables on them, what's left? Well, that leads to the *third* part of the interview, where it's time for you inspect your work surroundings. What does that entail? Well, that covers the main clinic you will be working in, any satellite facilities (make sure that you actually look at them, and not take them for granted), as well as any hospitals that you could be affiliated with. Depending on how the main interview goes and the length of time you have to visit, you may investigate the surrounding facilities during your initial visit or during a subsequent follow-up visit.

When it comes to satellite facilities, make sure you do a "test drive" between your main clinic and the outlying areas. Many physicians rightly claim that they do not generate income while driving. This can be true, and depending on the traveling distance and geography (rush hour traffic in Los Angeles, anyone?) it could really add up.

So what are some of the main areas of a practice to investigate?

Environment: Walk through the entire practice, including the staff lounge, physician offices, and the waiting room. Are they streamlined? Are they well maintained and clean?

Resources: Having enough staff and physical resources can really make your work environment wonderful—or not. Make sure the staff is large enough, morale is high, and that everyone appears to be getting along. It doesn't hurt to walk into the office, chat with the staff, and get a few impressions. Look into the exam rooms, chart areas, and supply cabinets and see if they're neat, stocked and well-organized. Again, no need to be overly obsessed to where you're raising eyebrows, but just get a general opinion.

Daily operations: How long do patients wait to be seen? How are they triaged, and what is the overall patient flow? How are calls handled during and after office hours? How is paperwork and billing handled? If not already transitioned, what, if any, plans for electronic billing and collections are in place? What about electronic charting? Believe it or not, the points previously mentioned are at the heart of how you and the members of your group are paid. Therefore, patient management, billing, collection, and charting systems must be up to par. Unfortunately, it is not uncommon to find deficiencies in these areas to some extent in many practices.

Meet the community: It is not unreasonable to meet with predecessors, other community physicians, pharmacists, hospital personnel, pharmaceutical representatives, or just about anyone with meaningful contact with the group. Most will be willing to comment and elaborate on their experience with the style, competence, and manner in which the group practices. Since they are not directly involved with the group, they may often be able to offer candid assessments that, through their comments, can help to establish a general community opinion of the practice.

FINANCIAL ANALYSIS

The *fourth* portion of the evaluation process is perhaps the most delicate and sensitive. It involves performing "financial due diligence," that is, a thoughtful financial analysis of the group you are considering to join. For obvious reasons this is not part of the initial evaluation process, but rather when serious negotiations are entered between you and the group. This topic is covered separately in Chapter 8.

After your visit is completed and you find that the practice's goals match your own, you will probably be happy in that environment. If so, don't hesitate to express your positive feelings. It is not only courteous, but professional to write a thank you note to the group after your visit. Additionally, after you have finished with the interview, it is important to collect your thoughts in order to compare this group and the offer to others. Refer to Appendix 3 for a sample chart that you can turn to when making your final decision.

7

UNDERSTANDING SALARY AND COMPENSATION ARRANGEMENTS

For most of us about to enter a professional relationship with a group or hospital, addressing the contract and its surrounding legal issues and complications is foreign territory. Although residencies are great in training physicians, there is little or no emphasis on contract negotiations. Add to this a myriad of financial options when it comes to salary, income, benefits, and the like, and it becomes easy to see why many new physicians end up with contracts they may regret. For instance, it is important to understand the difference between *salary* and *compensation package*. Salary is the up-front dollar figure, or wages paid on a regular basis, while compensation comprises retirement benefits, health insurance, bonuses, and the like.

Unfortunately, most physicians do not ask, or negotiate, the *compensation and benefits package*, which can often significantly eclipse a higher starting salary. The general attitude should be to approach contract negotiation and the economics of medicine with the same degree of sophistication as a physician approaches the practice of medicine.

Nonetheless, a detailed review by the physician as well as legal counsel is suggested, as entering into any agreement without such careful review is an open invitation to disaster. A caveat to this is to consider using an attorney in the state you are considering, versus your current state, if it differs. As state laws and customs vary, it may be beneficial to have an attorney from the area or, alternatively, one who is well versed in that particular specialty.

Although the vast majority of organizations that a young physician contemplates joining are not "out to get you," it is vitally important to understand certain terms, conditions, and methods of reimbursement in order to ensure that you receive a fair and beneficial contract that keeps both parties content. Read on to understand these various arrangements, some of which may not be in the contract, but perhaps can be negotiated. Also understand that this is an area of dynamic change and scrutiny from legal oversight, so be conscious of updates to various economic arrangements between yourself and a hospital or medical group. Other aspects discussed later may not pertain or be particularly appropriate for the position you are considering.

PHYSICIAN RECRUITMENT AGREEMENTS

It is becoming more common for hospitals to recruit physicians to particular medical communities using physician recruitment agreements (PRAs). What is a PRA? Well, it is essentially a way for a hospital to recruit a physician to a community with a (strictly) defined need or shortage for a particular physician specialty. For the physician, these agreements can *provide a guaranteed income for a designated time, cover relocation costs, offer a signing bonus,* and/or *relieve medical education debt.* For the hospital, it may be the only way to attract physicians where the demand far exceeds the supply (usually certain rural and urban areas).

There are usually two scenarios in which this occurs. In the first, the hospital helps a physician establish his or her own private practice. In this situation, be wary of the call schedule, as it will be up to you to arrange. Are there community physicians available and, importantly, willing to help the "new" guy (or gal) in town with taking call?

In the second PRA scenario, the employer, or medical group essentially forms an alliance with the local hospital to assist with its recruitment efforts. Depending on the arrangement, the group will either seek independent benefits from the PRA or retain/administer/distribute the PRA's economic benefits on behalf of the recruited physician. The PRA may also serve to thereby strengthen the relationship between a key physician group and the local hospital.

The following are some potential benefits of a PRA:

- Income guarantees
- Loan guarantees (know if you are getting a loan or an income guarantee and the difference between the two)
- Subsidized overhead expenses
- Reimbursement of relocation expenses
- Marketing allowances
- Financial assistance with practice startup
- Interest-free or low-interest loans
- Recruitment bonuses

It is important to know that these agreements are carefully regulated by government agencies, particularly by the federal antikickback statute. The main point of these restrictions is to prevent hospitals from "buying" or influencing a physician or group in exchange for referrals, goods, or services to a specific hospital or medical center. So, although hospital A may bring you into a particular community, there is no legal or other obligation keeping you from bringing patients and services to hospital B (although, off the record, it may be frowned upon).

The majority of these PRA agreements require the physician to serve the *community* (not the hospital; remember, that's illegal) for a minimum of 2 or 3 years. Any less, and there may be substantial financial penalties. Although the contract cannot restrict you to the recruiting hospital, they often do restrict you to a certain county or zip code area.

The total physician compensation may be subject to tax, fraud, abuse, and anti-self-referral laws. As such, compensation must be demonstrated to be a fair market value, or demonstrating reasonable compensation. Fair market value is determined by comparing the entire compensation package including all benefits, to industry standards relative to geography and specialty.

Because the laws concerning the antikickback statute are so broad, the Department of Health and Human Services has created certain "safe harbors" to define the terms surrounding PRAs. Although not complete, the main tenets surrounding PRAs are as follows. (For a complete list, go to: *http://bhpr.hrsa.gov/shortage/hpsaguidepc.htm*)

- The agreement must be set forth in writing, and you must understand every provision in the agreement before you execute it.
- The benefits are provided by the entity for a period not in excess of 3 years, and the terms cannot be renegotiated during this 3-year period in any substantial aspect.
- There is no requirement that the practitioner make referrals to, be in a position to make or influence referrals to, or otherwise generate business for the entity as a condition for receiving the benefits.
- The practitioner is not restricted from establishing staff privileges at, referring any services to, or otherwise generating any business for any other entity of his or her choosing.
- The payment or exchange of anything of value may not directly or indirectly benefit any person (other than the practitioner being recruited) or entity in a position to make or influence referrals to the entity providing the recruitment payments or benefits of items or services payable by a federal health care program.
- There is documented evidence of an objective need for the practitioner's services.

When the PRA agreement also involves employment by a private practice, ensure that there are no inconsistencies between the *two* contracts you will be signing. This is particularly important if neither the hospital nor the medical practice will execute (be bound by) the others' contract. Guess who will be left holding the (legal) bag. Don't let it be you.

An example of a potential legal and financial nightmare involving your obligations to both your medical practice contract and PRA contract is the following: Say that your medical group administers your PRA benefits (you forward all sums received under the agreement to the practice, who then pays you), but within the first year of a 3-year contract, terminates your services. They have collected and disbursed a portion of your PRA benefit, but owe nothing to the hospital providing the PRA in terms of obligations for the remaining portion of the contract. You are either now responsible for repaying a part or the entire amount of the PRA disbursement or, alternatively, continuing to practice in the hospital's service area. But if the group, which likely has a noncompete agreement with you, forces you out of the area, you could be left in a legal and financial mess. The best way to protect yourself from a scenario such as this is to have both the hospital and practice contracts reviewed by a contract lawyer for such discrepancies.

There are two main ways in which a PRA provides for a salary. The first is the *net income guarantee*. The second is in the form of an *income loan*. And yes, if you don't fulfill your end of the bargain, you could find yourself in the nasty situation of having to pay back a rather substantial loan. Most income guarantees are in effect for 1 year, with a 2- or 3-year residency requirement. This means that according to the contract, you are paid for 1 year, but are required to provide service to the area for 2 to 3 years.

The next thorn in most guarantees is that they usually pay for 1 year. Well, guess who is responsible for keeping the practice afloat for years two and three of the contract? You guessed it. That essentially gives you 1 *year* (assuming you started your own practice) to ramp up a practice large enough to support yourself and pay expenses. Depending on the circumstances, that may not be long enough, and you may find yourself struggling financially after the first year, as it is not unusual for the PRA salary to be rather generous, only to see a new physician's salary decrease, sometimes by 50%, in the second year. The major advice here is to resist the temptation to "live large" your first year; large house and car notes have no pity if your income tanks after your first year.

If expenses are separately paid in the contract, understand what expenses are paid and what are not. Typical expenses include rent, utilities, maintenance, employee salaries, office supplies, malpractice insurance, phones, accounting, etc. Personal salary, taxes, depreciation, and deferred compensation plans are usually not covered.

Speaking of taxes, it is important to find out if you will be responsible for taxes on the entire compensation package (if it includes expenses). Many packages provide a salary, as well as additional money for equipment. However, the entire funds may be paid to you as a disbursement, ultimately meaning that you could be paying income taxes on money that is used to pay for furniture, medical equipment, and the like. This could leave you with a sizeable tax burden.

Another way of looking at the income guarantee is to actually treat it as a type of subsidy. In this situation the hospital guarantees that you will have a certain take-home income. For example, let's say that you have an offer for an income guarantee of $120,000, or $10,000 a month. After celebrating with your friends, let's sit down and do the math. In month one, as you ramp up practice (billed receivables may be delayed for up to 90 days) let's say that you bring home $2,000 after expenses. Under the agreement, the hospital will "give" you $8,000 that month, so you take home a total of $10,000. 6 months into the practice, as you take home, say $6,000, the hospital is obligated to pay you $4,000. And the last month, as you make $10,000 in December, what do you get from the hospital? That's right—"zip" from the hospital. If you're lucky you'll get a card that says "Happy Holidays" and a pat on the back. Watch out what happens next, as some hospitals will entitle themselves to *any amount made over $10,000* during the contract, *or often for 2 to 3 months following the initial twelve*, as your reimbursements from the tail end of the contract come in. That's right, if you happen to make $12,000 your last month of the contract, *you owe them* $2,000. These features of a contract can vary, so read your contract and understand it thoroughly, asking for examples like the previous one. So in the end, although an income guarantee of $120,000 or greater can sound like a lot, the hospital's outlay can be substantially less. And they get to keep you around for 3 years.

A caveat of the income guarantee is that the hospital needs to have a defined, precise accounting of your (or your group's) billing, collection, and expenses. These are usually due within a certain number of days. Especially if you are with a group, it is important that you define the precise accounting mechanisms required by the hospital, and how your group intends to comply. Inattention on your groups' part can lead to loss or delay of your salary.

The second type of PRA involves providing a salary that is essentially treated as an income loan. In this arrangement, a certain amount is guaranteed to the physician. This interest-free loan is paid in installments, usually monthly or semimonthly. In the event you are starting your own practice, it is important to understand if practice expenses are to be taken out of this loan, or if expenses are included separately. In the latter situation, it is important to understand the extent of expenses covered, in detail. For example, a particular $300,000 offer may actually also cover business and operational expenses (overhead). Remember that overhead usually averages 50%. After paying that, the offer may really turn into $150,000. Remember, as most offers extend the loan for year one of the practice, it is your responsibility to develop a practice that covers expenses and generates income for years two and three of the contract, and beyond. A caveat of this arrangement is that a *physician's salary can plummet* after the first year. Remember that you must become financially viable by the end of 1 year, if practicing on your own.

The next aspect of a PRA is to understand how the income guarantee or loan is forgiven. This is contingent upon your remaining within the hospital's service area (note that this does not imply having to stay with a particular practice or group). The guarantee, or loan, should be forgiven incrementally, that is, for every month or year of service a portion of the total guarantee is forgiven. Failure to complete the contract will require that a *portion or total amount of the loan be paid back.*

Although unexpected and unwished, it is also important to understand the ramifications of repayment in the circumstance of disability. Your private employment agreement should cover short- and or long-term disability. It is important to make sure that you are protected from repayment obligations as to the PRA if you become permanently disabled.

On a final note, PRAs may dictate the number of hours or days worked per day, week, or month. In addition, vacation time may be stipulated. Know and understand these terms.

Although there are many aspects of the PRA that may appear daunting or otherwise not in your favor, it is important to understand that the

PRA has also emerged as an excellent tool, and often a financially reward-ing option for a physician to join a particular medical group or community. Understand that many facets of the PRA are negotiable, and it is possible, with diligence and care to design a mutually beneficial contract.

COMPENSATION BASED ON PRODUCTIVITY

In this setup, the physician is usually paid a set amount of his or her prior months' charges, minus adjustments. These adjustments will typically include overhead costs, as well as adjusting for the collection percentage rate. In many incentive-based plans, quality-control contingencies will be in place, such as patient satisfaction scoring. This intends to prevent increasing productivity in the face of decreased quality of care. For exam-ple, say a physician bills for $10,000 in a given month. Subtract the col-lection rate, say 60%. That leaves $6,000 "collected". From this, subtract a 50% overhead, leaving $3,000, which goes to the physician. In some sit-uations, a group may bill for charges on a current basis and await collec-tion, which can be an average of 60 to 90 days. In this scenario, payment can be delayed 60 to 90 days. For example, March's salary is based on col-lections from January. This can have a significant impact on the first year's income and bonus. Variations are common, so understand the specifics of your particular contract.

COMPENSATION BASED ON GROUP OR PHYSICIAN NET INCOME

Net income is defined as that amount remaining after deduction or pay-ment of *all* practice expenses. In this arrangement, the physician's income can be reflected as a percentage of the net income he or she brings in to the group, or as an evenly divided amount of net income to the group. Although it may sound simple, the main issue with this setup is that what defines income and expenses for a group may be subject to dispute. What if certain members of a group are part of separate ventures? Which costs should be borne by the group, and which by individuals? Although equal income distribution plans can placate certain disputes, disparate physician productivity and expenses can also cause their unique problems.

FORMULA-BASED COMPENSATION

A variety of formulas may be utilized, which may include multiple factors in calculation. Each may be given a certain weight, points, or percentage in calculating salary. These may involve productivity, board certification, administrative roles, new patients, referral sources, teaching or research activities, goodwill, stock ownership, and longevity in the practice (make sure there is a maximum of points per year a doctor can earn).

It is important that you have a concept of what you expect to earn in your first year, 3- to 5-year range, and longer term. Ask for examples of calculations, and what partners in the practice make. As such formulas can be complicated, find out the history and any problems with their formula-based compensation plan and any significant changes made.

Finally, make sure the details of the calculation and any examples are explicitly outlined in the contract. Also understand how and why a compensation formula can change. It is not unusual to find situations where you are hired and promised one formula, only to find that it changes during, or after you become a partner.

FIXED SALARY

Many physicians are paid a fixed-base salary. It is important to understand the amount and frequency (monthly, bimonthly, etc.) of payments, as well as what deductions are made. Also investigate cost-of-living adjustments. If your salary does not adjust for inflation (lately 3% per year on average), your effective salary may actually be reduced over time.

Although many salary arrangements may be financially lucrative, those offered a low base salary may want to push for a high level of benefits. This includes timing and evaluations for future raises, retirement benefits, health insurance, and the like. In this vein, look at your salary as part of the total *compensation* package.

RELATIVE VALUE UNIT-BASED SALARY

The relative value unit (RVU) concept was introduced by the Centers for Medicare & Medicaid Services (CMS) in 1991. This structure may be found in large, or managed-care groups. RVUs are blinded to reimbursement, collections, and the like. Instead, they assign a certain value to patient encounters and procedures. This may be beneficial for physicians who do a fair amount of work, which is not reflected in billing or collections. This includes those who see a large number of Medicaid or capitated patients. In this model, salary can be indexed to RVU production based on published tables linking RVU by geography, specialty, and other factors.

BONUSES

When it comes to bonuses, it may not be unreasonable to ask for a history of bonuses within the group. That way, you have an understanding that what you are being offered is not a "pie in the sky" that you are unlikely to attain. Second, as the bonus structure may be complex, make sure that the definitions and methodology for calculation are clear to both parties. You may even request a sample calculation to be included. In the event of dispute, the contract serves as a reference for clarification.

Bonuses may be paid when the physician meets certain target gross production or collection targets. The distinction between collection-based and production-based formulas should be made clear in the contract. If ancillary services or physician extenders are utilized, know if those collections and productions are included (usually not).

Collection-Based Bonus

The most common method for calculating a bonus is to pay a percentage of the physician's collections over a specified amount. The "kick-in" point for the bonus structure, as well as percentage paid, are commonly negotiable. An example of this is to pay 25% of collections made over

$10,000 in a month. If you brought in $20,000 that month, or $10,000 over the kick-in point, you would get $2,500, or 25% of the amount made above and beyond your bonus set point.

Production-Based Bonus

A method similar to that for compensation-based bonus is used for production-based bonus, with the exception of how production is calculated. Production usually includes all charges in a given period, as recorded on the charge slips or superbills, adjusted by certain contractual allowances. These allowances account from the difference between amount billed and the fees actually charged to Medicare, managed care arrangements, or from other discounted fees.

RVU-Based Bonus

As discussed in the income section, here RVUs are used to calculate a bonus. A threshold RVU number is established, with a dollar figure attached to an established set of benchmarks for production above and beyond a certain RVU.

SPECIAL CONSIDERATIONS FOR THOSE CONSIDERING A CAREER IN ACADEMIA

Given that many academic programs are becoming more and more geared toward clinical productivity, it is important for a prospective individual to investigate the taxation structure of the group practice and understand how incentives can be reached. Specifically, most academic physicians tend to be salaried to some extent. The base salary and any bonuses tend to be dependant on clinical productivity above and beyond the bottom line. In order the reach the bottom line, the income must pass through the institution's taxation system. That is to say, for every dollar of clinical productivity an academic physician makes, a certain proportion is designated for administrative support staff, such as secretarial support and office overhead. Frequently after that, several other entities may apply taxes to the bottom line. Often there is a Dean's tax applied by the Dean of the institution. Also, the overseeing department and/or division may assess a tax on the productivity. There may be other taxes depending on the institutional structure. Sometimes, these taxes are the means by which the academic structure survives. The important issue is to understand the tax and incentive structure and make sure that it ultimately provides sufficient incentive for financial growth and does not simply support the more senior and higher ranking members of the institution. These financial arrangements vary significantly, and the percentage of salary given to the overhead of an academic practice can be substantial.

NOTE ON ANCILLARY REVENUE STREAMS

As reimbursement continues to be under pressure, many physicians augment their income from ancillary revenue streams. This ancillary revenue may come from additional laboratory or radiology services, ambulatory surgical centers, dialysis centers, mobile lithotripters, bone densitometry testing, and such. It is important to clarify whether you will be able to partake in revenue generated from these sources, especially since you will likely be contributing clinical volume to these profit centers within the group. In most situations, profit sharing from these areas may be limited or restricted until you become a full partner in the practice. Although this is not unreasonable while you are employed, it is important to have in writing what the terms and conditions are for vesting in shares of ancillary ventures once you become a partner. The reason for this is that you do not want to be in a situation where you find that the terms, amounts, or even eligibility to become a shareholder in an ancillary venture are different from those discussed when being initially recruited to the practice,. There are many stories of young physicians being courted to a practice with the lure of additional revenue streams, only to find that they are denied a buy-in, or that the terms are unreasonably prohibitive. To reiterate, *include future and current buy-in provisions to ancillary ventures in your contract.*

OVERVIEW OF EXPENSE STRUCTURE

Although expense calculation was incorporated into some of the salary structure discussed earlier, it is broken down separately here, into the major methods utilized:

Direct Costs

Each physician is liable for the expenses incurred by that individual. This allows for flexibility in tailoring expenditure to individual practice style, equipment, personnel, etc.

Indirect Costs

Overhead costs including rent, utilities, maintenance, and the like are charged based on square footage utilized in that part of the practice.

Equal Assessment

Expenses are deducted from gross revenue, and net income is then divided equally among physicians. The issue here is a perceived inequality between resource utilization and productivity between physicians. Look into any history of problems in this expense structure and methods for addressing issues that may come up.

Expenses as a Percentage of Productivity

In this model, each physician is charged for expenses at the same rate that he or she generates income. For example, if a doctor earns 20% of the group's income, he or she will be responsible for 20% of the expenses.

8

FINANCIAL DUE DILIGENCE: INVESTIGATING THE PRACTICE

Once you have gone through the proper evaluation of a group, and are seriously considering it among your top choices, it is important that you get an idea of the groups' finances. Based on the type of practice arrangement you are considering joining, different aspects of this chapter may or may not be relevant to you.

If you are about to join the Veteran's Administration system, a detailed financial analysis is obviously not warranted. However, even if you are joining an academic or institutional group, being oblivious to finances can hurt you. Even the academic world, once sheltered from the bane of strict financial accountability, is being increasingly pressured to show productivity and financial responsibility. Inadvertently joining an academic group with significant financial issues could possibly jeopardize your budding career. So, regardless of your career choice in medicine, it pays to have a basic understanding of financial terms that you may encounter, which ultimately can leave you less vulnerable in the negotiation and contract phases.

The first questions that often arise when it comes to investigating a groups' finances are: What is appropriate, and how much information am I entitled to ask for and receive? Many new physicians emerging from residency and meeting with new employers may feel obviously reluctant to request sensitive information on a groups' financial performance. But is it inappropriate? Well, to look at it this way, joining a medical practice can be considered a major investment of yourself, your career, and training. The potential risks and rewards of this investment are too great to ignore. Just as any investment in a house, it requires proper due diligence. Indeed, most proper employers should view the request for information as appropriate and as a sign of your diligence and professionalism. *Any unwarranted or excessive hostility or inability to produce basic information or documents should raise a red flag.*

That said, how much information you seek and receive, depends on your comfort level with a particular group. Remember, it is your right to ask such information. The key issues to look out for are glossed over answers such as, "The numbers look great for this year," and "I wouldn't worry about the future numbers...You'll do great as a partner" on one extreme, to putting up a wall on the other, "We don't discuss our numbers with anyone who isn't a partner with the group." Instead, you want thoughtful and honest numbers. A group that seems honest but can't put together the numbers or answers for you may indicate messy (not dishonest) accounting, but just the same raises a red flag.

To follow is a list of potential information to obtain from a group. The most common scenarios and issues encountered will be listed earlier, with more specific or arcane issues a bit further down. Depending on how financially savvy you may be, it helps to enlist an accountant or experienced physician to help you tease through the information and understand what is within a normal range, and what numbers generate cause for concern. *Remember, when it comes to the contract, don't assume. If it's not written down, it doesn't exist.*

- The groups' overhead-to-revenue ratio

This is a key number to get. If you need to get one number, obtain this one. It is a key indicator of how the overall practice is managed. Most groups will readily divulge this information without problems. Remember, the expenses **generally** should not exceed 50% of the revenue, and the lower, the better.

- Current income distribution plan

Also investigate problems, past history, and anticipated changes. This varies between groups and specialties. Look for a plan that is fair and well accepted by the partners, as this can often be a great source of conflict within a group. Are salaries divided evenly or based on productivity? Most plans have a basis in one or the other.

- Realistic production rate that can be achieved by the candidate by the end of the first year

A critical question. If the opening salary is high, can you sustain it? And if it is lower than average, is there a potential upside in the long term?

- Group outlook and goals

The group should be able to state clearly plans for where it wants to be in the 1-, 3-, and 5-year time span. First, see if they actually have a plan. If they seem flustered, because they are actually figuring it out as they speak to you, be aware of a lack of group cohesion and communication. Overall, you should be left confident that the group's goals are realistic, achievable, and in line with your own expectations.

- Anticipated major capital projects and costs in the next 3 to 5 years

Don't get caught off guard that they intend to build a brand new clinic in 2 years. Although you may stand to gain from it, you'll also be paying for it.

- Payor mix for the last 3 to 5 years

Many practitioners will seek a larger population with private insurance. Specifically, you will also want to get an idea of what reimbursement rates are. "1.0" means that insurance contracts are paying Medicare index rates. "1.5," which is high, or 1.5 times Medicare rates, are an example of payments in less competitive or rural areas. Rates such as "0.8," or less than Medicare, are often seen in highly competitive areas or fields with high managed-care penetration. Medicare as a percentage of the practice varies with your specialty. Generally, most providers want to minimize Medicaid or free-care patients. These numbers also vary significantly based on the market you practice in. You will need to speak to several physicians to get an idea of what the norms for a particular field and geography are.

- Management (large groups)

How is the group managed? If there is a full-time administrator, does he or she demonstrate competence? Does he or she have the support of office and physician staff? Is this person someone you can work with (you will spend a lot of time with this person)? Good management is often at the root of group profitability.

- Existing and anticipated provider contracts

Usually one or two plans will provide a large percentage of patients. Focus your investigation on these companies and contracts.

  o   Financial condition
  o   Number of enrollees
  o   Type of plans
  o   Terms of contract (fee schedule, ways to modify fees)
  o   Reimbursement methods
  o   Termination provisions (getting out of bad contracts)
  o   Extent of capitated contracts (present risk to group)

- Retirement policy

Is there one? How is it funded? More importantly, since you're not the one retiring yet, how do the senior-most partners retire? Why does that affect you? Senior partners may often be "bought out" of their stake in the clinic. Find out what this includes, as some policies involve paying out their stake in the fixed assets, as well as a certain amount of goodwill. Just make sure you're not bearing an unreasonable or unfair burden in funding someone else's golden parachute.

- Balance sheet, including profit and loss statements for the last 3 to 5 years; include revenue sources (ie, ancillary and other services)

If there are several outlying offices, are they equally busy, or is there one that is consistently poorly performing? Guess who could end up there. If there are partnerships involving endoscopy suites, surgical centers, dialysis centers, labs, etc., how do they perform?

- Receivables history

Most insurance plans are obligated to pay groups within 90 days. You want to look out for a long history of delinquent payments, nonpayments, or poor collection history. This may mean the group is not aggressive enough with collections, or simply working with poor contracts and insurance carriers.

- Operating and capital budgets

Make sure that you are dealing with a streamlined operation without excess frills or allowances.

- Overall practice debt

Understand why the debt was incurred, interest rates, and repayment plans. High debt? No good.

- o   3- to 5-year history; ratio to gross revenue
- o   Short- and long-term debt
- o   Reasons for each loan
- o   Anticipated near-term debt
- o   Repayment history and schedules

- The groups' physician productivity summary

Are all physicians equally productive, or are there significant differences? Large differences can sometimes cause trouble within a group.

- o   3- to 5-year history
- o   By specialty (if multispecialty)
- o   By physician

9

NEGOTIATING A FAIR AND PROPER CONTRACT

Understand that although this text attempts to cover most salient points, complex state and federal statutes and regulations are not covered. Some of the terms and provisions may be inapplicable or inappropriate or not sufficiently detailed. Independent contractor agreements and employee–shareholder and other professional corporation arrangements are beyond the scope of this text. In a similar vein, although addressed in part, certain legal relationships are based on contract, employment, tax, and government laws that are individualized and reflect specific employment situations. As such, this manual does not constitute legal advice, and does not substitute for individualized, in-depth analysis by a legal expert.

As the face of health care continues to change, more and more young physicians are finding themselves employed. Whether this is via a traditional medical group practice or another entity, physicians are increasingly covered by employment contracts. Thus, it is important that you have at least a basic understanding of terminology and the major elements of most physician employment agreements.

The negotiation process can be intimidating, especially to a young physician just out of training. Just as knowledge can make a good physician better, having a basic knowledge of the terms and nature of contract negotiation can make you a more adept negotiator and keep you out of trouble and in a long-term relationship that you will enjoy. If that sounds a bit like marriage, you're right. That brings up another point. If appropriate, involve your spouse in the negotiation process. If one is to be happy, both need to be happy!

The law assumes that when you sign a contract, that you have agreed to all of the terms. It does not protect you from making a bad deal, or an unfair agreement. Ignorance of the law doesn't protect you in the event that things go sour. Therefore, involving an attorney experienced in health care law and contracts is important. The cost may be a few to several hundred dollars, but may turn out to be minute when you compare it to the thousands of dollars lost in fighting a bad contract or job situation.

Utilizing a lawyer also needs to be handled with tact. Although the contract should be thoroughly evaluated by a lawyer, "aggressive" negotiation with a lawyer (it's not unheard of to use a lawyer to negotiate the contract on a physician's behalf, or to bring a lawyer to a negotiation session) can be contentious and off-putting to a group. Use tact and common sense, but always have a lawyer covering you in the background.

Just as athletes with special talents have formidable power at the negotiation table, it is important that you understand your specific talents that give you additional leverage. You're not likely to get a multimillion-multiyear contract, but it does help. Points that strengthen your case include having fellowship training and subspecialty interests, speaking certain languages, being a native of a certain area, or belonging to a certain ethnic group that may relate to a particular patient population.

Finally, it is important to understand that the endpoint of your negotiations is to be a content, functional part of a group or organization. Sure, it's important to be paid (just not taken advantage of), but also understand that it is important to treat the negotiation process as the beginning of a relationship with the group. As such, negotiations should not be approached in a hostile manner, and it is key to come prepared with an understanding of which areas you are prepared to compromise on, and "leave things on the table," and which areas are important in order for you to be content with the relationship. Remember, the goal of this process is for you to become a partner and not squeeze the group out of every last dollar (unless it really is). Again, remember that not all aspects of contracts described later in the chapter will apply to everyone. For example, it is rare for physicians in the government sector to receive bonus compensation.

Before we start dissecting the main components of the contract, we'll cover some main pitfalls and issues regarding contracts:

1. *Negotiate, negotiate, negotiate.*

    Without sounding repetitive, look at the original contract as a rough draft. Remember that most terminology is there to protect the employer's interests, and not your own. Look out for yourself, and remember that all aspects of the contract, and not just salary, are negotiable. Lay your job offers side by side and analyze them for deal breakers. Don't sign a contract that you're unhappy with, in the hope that you can negotiate more favorable terms after you've been with the practice for a while. Remember that at the outset of negotiations, when the practice wants to hire you, you're negotiating from a position of strength. A year or two later into practice, unless you become one of the practice's superstars, you'll have far less bargaining power.

2. *Get it in writing.*

    It is not unusual for a group to rely on verbal assurances, "We've always done it that way," and customary practices. Administrators, partners, and department heads change frequently. Having everything in writing is the safest way to keep from being sorry later, and allows for the agreement to survive any changes in the group.

3. *Take time.*

    Insist on enough time to thoroughly consider the contract. Don't feel rushed (even if you are), and try not to succumb to pressure tactics from a recruiter or the employer. That may be a red flag, if anything.

4. *Don't assume.*

    If you don't understand something in a contract, have it explained. Don't assume that it's just harmless wording. Instead, have it explained and possibly reworded. You'll often find that the group itself has a tough time explaining "legalese." Don't sign anything that you don't understand, and don't be embarrassed to ask. You are a doctor after all, and not a legal professional.

5. *Attach it.*

    Make sure all external references to attachments, documents, and exhibits are included with the contract (often referred to as incorporation by reference).

For the sake of (relative) simplicity, we will break the contract down into three sections. The first will address *compensation*. Compensation and bonus structure are covered in greater depth elsewhere in the text. The second part will look into the *terms of employment*. The third addresses *termination*.

PART I: COMPENSATION

The first part of the contract involves *compensation*. What is that? Well, that includes salary, bonus, insurance premiums, pension and retirement plans, expense accounts, professional dues, journal subscriptions, hospital staff fees, moving costs, continuing medical education (CME) expense reimbursement, loans, research stipends, and honoraria. Each is covered separately in detail later.

Salary

Most practices will usually guarantee a certain salary during the early portion of employment. Since billing and collecting are usually delayed by as long as 90 days, and there is certain time associated with building a practice, the practice usually will need to support the new recruit's salary. The salary range will vary greatly depending on practice location, specialty, years of training, and demand, to name a few. Although the tables provided in the text will give you an estimated idea, speaking to local colleagues is the best way to get a "real time" idea of fair and reasonable salaries for your position.

After an initial period, compensation may shift in the direction of a productivity-based salary. If the salary is to be tied to productivity, consider how patients will be allocated in the group. It is not unheard of to find the new physician "dumped on"; getting all Medicare/Medicaid, indigent patients, and the like, while senior partners "cherry-pick" the patient load.

Bonus

The first type of bonus is a sign-on incentive. A sign-on bonus may or may not be an option, depending largely on the demand in your particular field and area.

The second is tied to productivity. This rewards a physician for building a practice that is greater than expected for the given salary. A well-negotiated incentive plan can actually be more important than salary, as it rewards hard work and can greatly supplement one's salary. If the bonus is tied to multiple factors, ensure that the bonus is tied to factors within your control, such as the money you bring in, patient load, expenses, etc. The main points surrounding a bonus structure include the magic number above which a bonus is applicable; second, how much is paid above that number, and third, any additional formulas or factors such as patient satisfaction scores or patient volume, as discussed earlier.

To give an example, say a physician is paid a $100,000 salary. Estimating a 50% expense or overhead ratio, that means that $200,000 of revenue would have to be brought in. Any amount above that usually goes back to the practice (they make money off the recruit). In a negotiated bonus structure, you would claim a certain percentage (negotiated) above that designated dollar figure. That percentage can range from a few percent to 100%, although typically between 40 to 80%. The group may claim expenses associated with hiring the new physician to justify holding onto some of the additional revenue generated by the new recruit.

An important point about negotiated bonuses is that they are unlikely to be seen during your first year of practice, as you ramp-up. Instead, they become more valuable with longer contracts, or with contracts with a longer (3 year) time to partnership.

The third aspect of bonus structure is subjective. By its very nature, they are often vague and variable. In some group structures where all partners are paid equally, for instance, any operating revenue at the end of the month or year, after expenses are paid, may be doled out as a bonus. In other instances, partners may subjectively feel that you have worked hard and made a great impression in the community, and deserve a bonus.

Depending on the structure and culture of a group, bonuses may or may not exist. In comparison, other complex bonus structures may exist. Just understand how they work, and don't hesitate to draw up theoretical numbers.

Insurance Coverage

There are four main types of insurance premiums that practices may typically provide for an entering physician. Again, benefits are variable, and some, all, or none can be expected depending on each circumstance. The main point is to inquire if you do not see certain benefits. Finally, if the employer is paying less than the full premium on any of the policies, ensure that the amount or percentage each party is responsible for is noted.

HEALTH INSURANCE   This is one of the most important, and usually covered, benefits. It is important that coverage extends not only to the new physician, but the family as well. Make sure of the degree that premiums are paid (usually entirely), and the extent of coverage and copays.

DISABILITY INSURANCE   This is often provided by the group as well. Investigate the extent and type of coverage. Find out if the policy is "own occupation" or not. This type of policy is better, as it covers you in the event you cannot practice medicine *in your own specialty*. An example of this is a disabled surgeon who elects to do insurance physicals to supplement income. An "own occupation" policy allows this, and continues to pay; newer policies without this exclusion will treat this as physician income, and will partially or fully deduct this income. Some will even extend this to *any* income generated, even if you decide to start a lawn-mowing service. Also beware of a statute of limitation, that is, where the "own occupation" only extends a defined (3 to 5 year) period after the injury.

The second aspect of disability insurance is taxes: who pays them, and how that affects compensation under the policy. Simply, if you pay taxes on the policy, any pay-out will be tax-free, the benefits of which can be quite significant. However, if your group pays your disability premiums (a tax-free benefit to you, since it is taken out of your salary), you will end up paying taxes on any compensation from the policy. A way around this is to ask for additional salary compensation, and pay for the disability premiums for yourself.

Last, the disability insurance provided to you by the practice is often referred to as "group coverage." Depending on your circumstances, it is highly recommended that you look into carrying your own individual policy. If you are currently in residency, rates may be somewhat lower, and worth looking into. The benefits of an individual policy are that they are portable. This means that no matter what your job situation is, health circumstances are, etc., as long as you pay premiums, you will have coverage.

The new reality is that most physicians do not stay at one position their entire careers. This means that you will be dependent on your next group's coverage (or lack thereof). What happens as insurance policy coverage and restrictions continue to become more limited over time? What happens if you develop hypertension or diabetes in the interim? Or hepatitis from a needlestick?

A benefit of establishing individual disability coverage early in your career is that you lock in rates at an earlier age. As you get older, establishing coverage goes up. Premiums established at age 29 are significantly less than those starting at age 39 or 49. Add to that features such as "own occupation," and policies are getting harder and more expensive to find. Furthermore, adding group coverage on top of individual coverage usually results in a greater overall benefit, versus having preexisting group coverage, and then adding individual coverage. Details of these policies are intricate and vary widely. It is important that you contact a reliable policy agent who explains each policy in an understandable and thorough manner.

MALPRACTICE INSURANCE AND TAIL COVERAGE   This type of insurance is important and its provision varies depending on geography and specialty. In most cases, you will want to insist on coverage by the group. Indeed, most groups cover malpractice as part of the agreement. Make sure that yours does, and that you do not pay taxes on this benefit. Make sure that the coverage and policy limits are adequate based on your states' laws.

There are two main types of policies:

- *Occurrence Policy.*
  This policy covers malpractice events that happened during the policy period, regardless of the date of discovery or when the claim is filed.

For example, if a patient undergoes a hernia repair that fails years later, any action taken would be covered, whether the physician is still with the same insurance carrier or not. Since claims are effectively covered for the lifetime of the patient or occurrence, these policies tend to be more expensive.

- *Claims-Made Policy.*

This policy covers incidents that take place and are filed during the coverage period. It is usually cheaper for new physicians (25% less than a similar occurrence policy), as there is lower "exposure" (you have few, if any patients that could potentially sue you). Over time the pool of potential claimants increases and stabilizes (usually 5 years), allowing the insurance premium to stabilize as well. The rates may approximate an occurrence policy at this point.

What is tail coverage? Briefly, most practices provide a claims-made policy that protects the policyholder from claims for acts that occur and are reported to the insurer while the policy is in force. For example, say you leave California to set up a practice in New York. What happens to the patients you took care of in California under your old policy? This is where tail coverage comes in—it covers you for events and suits that occur after your claims-made policy ends.

Find out who covers tail coverage. Often, it will be you. Find out what happens when you become a partner. It is not unreasonable to share the costs, or have them covered entirely after partnership, as you may be able to assert that tail coverage deals with services and procedures you performed while still a revenue-generating member of the group. Also make the distinction between who pays tail coverage if you leave the group, and who pays if you are terminated by the group. Tail coverage in certain states can be as much as 100 to 150% of a claims-made policy, sometimes upwards of $50,000. *This can become an invisible leash to your group, making it financially impossible for you to leave.*

LIFE INSURANCE   Life insurance is probably the least important compared to the policies described earlier. Standard inclusion of life insurance is widely variable in most contracts, and not frequently seen. Most physicians will elect to carry a personal policy. Negotiating for this in your contract, if not present, is of minimal benefit.

Retirement or Pension Plans

Most practices will offer a standard tax-deferred retirement or pension plan. This is usually a standard type of plan offered to all physician-employees, and it is usually unreasonable to negotiate for benefits above and beyond that received by others in the group. Do understand the terms and nature of the plan. This includes maximum contribution (subject to federal guidelines), contribution matching, if any, and the portfolio of investment options. Certain profit-sharing plans may also be included, but make sure the details are understood.

Fringe Benefits

These are usually negotiable to a variable extent. Understand your limits, and those of the group. Remember that your goal is partnership, not to extract every last bit of money (and perhaps goodwill) from the group. Benefits to look into include expense accounts (say you have to do a fair amount of traveling between clinics and hospitals), student loan repayment (variable, and more common in hospital-sponsored offers), professional society dues, journal subscriptions, hospital staff fees (all usually covered), moving costs, CME reimbursement, CME time, and vacation.

MOVING Depending on the extent of the contract and negotiations, moving expenses can involve the expense of moving household items, transportation of the physician and family, packing/unpacking costs, moving insurance, storage costs, and temporary living expenses. Understand the extent to which moving expenses are covered. Additionally, agreements will also often stipulate that if the contract is terminated within a certain period (often 1 year), a portion (prorated) or the entire moving stipend will be repaid to the group.

HOUSING AND RELATED MATTERS Some large groups may additionally provide housing-related benefits. This can include expenses of selling the physician's existing home, house-hunting expenses in the new area, and closing costs. Additionally, some of the largest groups, especially those in expensive housing markets, can offer help with down payments or low-interest mortgage assistance. Understand the details of such agreements as well as the conditions relating to termination of the contract. Beware that large loans such as mortgages can often tie one to a group in the event the relationship sours. This can leave you in the position of a large repayment to the organization in order to terminate the contract.

VACATION AND SICK LEAVE   The contract should spell out the number of paid vacation days, and whether or not they may be carried over. The same should be detailed in regard to CME days. In some cases, vacation and CME time are lumped together; in others they are separated. Know the difference. Sick leave is usually cumulative, often to a total of 90 days, which coincides with the standard waiting period prior to being eligible for disability payments.

STUDENT LOAN PAYMENTS   As graduating new-physician debt gets larger and larger, this can be an important benefit. Understand that an employer's payment of student loans is still taxable to the employee. Payments are usually based on anniversary dates of the contract and are often not paid in a lump sum manner. This may require you to continue with monthly payments.

DUES AND LICENSES   The physician's membership in national, state, county, and specialty medical societies is an important benefit usually covered by most groups. Most also include hospital medical staff dues. As most contracts state that your employment is contingent on such memberships, insist that these dues are paid on your behalf.

Outside Income Policy

Covered here are speaking honorariums, teaching, writing, directorships, inventions, and intellectual property. Although most physicians do not moonlight at this point, some do, and you need to find out the restrictions. It may not be unusual for a group to be entitled to all or part of these proceeds. The contract should therefore stipulate to whom compensation from such activities belong.

PART II: TERMS OF EMPLOYMENT

Duration of Employment

The terms of employment begin with the duration that the contract remains in force. Unless otherwise specified, most contracts are terminable at will, meaning that either party can terminate the relationship at any time. Therefore, it is usually prudent for the contract to specify a fixed term. Ensure that any multiyear contract makes allowances for a cost-of-living increase; otherwise effective income may actually decrease over time.

In most situations, the agreement is for one, two, or 3 years. Most modern contracts should offer partnership within one to 2 years. For the 1 year, most groups subsidize the new partner as he or she ramps up the practice. Once you are essentially able to sustain yourself (1 to 2 years) partnership is appropriate. This also gives the group a "buffer" period to evaluate you as an individual and as a physician. It also gives you sufficient time to evaluate the practice as a long-term relationship. Partnership tracks greater than 2 years should be a point of negotiation, as longer periods are difficult to justify, and often allow the group to profit from the new physician. It happens.

Scope of Physician's Duties

This part of the contract will detail the physician's responsibilities. This includes both medical and administrative tasks. This can sometimes be in the form of a job description. Depending on the size and structure of the organization, administrative tasks may be as basic as maintaining medical records and billing, to more complex duties such as sitting on medical review panels, compulsory medical staff meetings, teaching, and the like. If these additional tasks are required, make note of the anticipated time and frequency, as well as any additional compensation if appropriate. Some contracts may specify administrative time such as a half-day per week, free from appointments, to address such duties.

Several other questions and issues can be brought up in this section. If a physician has subspecialty or fellowship training, will there be priority

.n assignment of relevant cases? If this is an issue, it should be addressed here. If salary is tied to productivity, is there a promise of a certain amount of work? If there are several locations to the practice, it may be prudent to note the main site of practice, and any possible rotation and travel schedules.

Partnership and Buy-In/Buy-Out Formula

For most individuals, employment arrangements are entered with an eye toward partnership or ownership. A correlate of employment as discussed earlier, the partnership track should begin within 1 to 2 years at best, upon starting employment. Partnership usually entails a certain cost, but there is no set formula. Look closely at what the buy-in includes, or restated, what you actually buy into. Does it include all assets, including investments? Salary structure usually changes as well, and often becomes performance based. Know the details.

A key point not to forget is that just as becoming a partner has a great potential "upside," *you also buy into the risk and liability of the group.* If there are Medicare billing issues or pending litigation against the group as a whole, you may be buying into that as well.

You will want to know what your buy in/out points are in detail, and also that of the last few partners. It is important to find out the latter, as the rules may change in the middle of the game. This may create tension and unfair advantages or disadvantages. Why did Dr. X "get in" for $10,000 after 1 year, and now you have to pony up $50,000 after 3 years? This needs to be strictly defined and written in the contract. It is not unusual to find doctors that are promised one deal and find a very different, worse arrangement later.

It is also critical to find out how the buy-in amount is calculated. It is typical to have an inventory of the "hard" assets of the group (computers, equipment, buildings, etc.) and divide it evenly. This is fair, but have a definition of how this will be calculated, and what it includes ahead of time. Accounts receivables, equipment, supply inventory, office buildings, real estate, and liabilities should all be detailed. Should the receptionist's 10-year-old desk be valued at $2,000? Make sure depreciated values are part of the calculation.

If the buy-in specifies that you are purchasing assets versus stock, know the difference. Assets are just that, while purchase of stock implies assumption of liability as well.

Another component of the buy-in may involve indexing the value of a practice to a percentage of the average taken of the groups' last 3- to 5-year financial "snapshot." This could involve gross revenue, net revenue, or a host of other calculations. The important thing to realize is that it doesn't take a genius to know that in this day and age, reimbursements can change overnight. That means a group's running 3- to 5-year averages could have little bearing on its future prospects.

The next portion of the buy-in is more complicated. That involves a value for goodwill. And no, it's not your goodwill. Goodwill entails the subjective value of a practice, which is often tied to the reputation and skill of the group. An established 30-year practice that is well known has a degree of goodwill with its patients, referring physicians, and community. A new practice and physician have little, if any.

The problem with goodwill is that it is hard to define and quantify. As traditional medicine has shifted to capitated and other managed care plans, patients are often forced to trade physician-based loyalty to that based on participation in managed care plans. Thus it is not unreasonable to see a group's goodwill disappearing overnight. Although difficult, try to avoid or minimize goodwill as part of your buy-in. Here's an example of how you can be burned on this: Say you paid $25,000 for hard assets, and $25,000 for goodwill. The next year your group is investigated, and closed down for Medicare fraud. You may be able to recoup part of your investment by selling the fixed assets, but you will never recover the goodwill, which in this case, was bad will.

If a goodwill valuation is unavoidable, make sure that the range of valuation is based on careful market conditions over the next several years. For most newly trained physicians, this is next to impossible to judge. To minimize grossly overpaying, or be taken advantage of, it may be wise to involve an attorney or financial advisor skilled in such matters to assist with proper valuation of a practice. It is not unusual to find groups that estimate goodwill without a concrete basis for such numbers.

In summary, goodwill valuations were quite common 5 to 10 years ago, but are becoming less prevalent as managed care and other constraints have led to uncertainties regarding ongoing practice value. Adopting a "it's only worth what *you* put into it" strategy may be prudent.

NO PARTNERSHIP OPPORTUNITY?   For those employed by hospitals, certain institutions, or other nonphysician employers, it may not be an option to establish an ownership or equity interest in the group. In these situations, it is prudent to involve language in the contract to allow for adjustments in salary and/or benefits based on time, periodic evaluation of performance, or other benchmarks.

Financing

Although the buy-in amount has reduced as goodwill values have been dropped or decreased, the amount itself is usually tens of thousands of dollars. Most groups will and should allow for payment (without interest) over a fixed number of years.

Call Coverage

You can bet that the partners of the practice you are considering to join are eagerly awaiting your arrival, if only because they get to add you to the call rotation. Just ensure that this is fair to an extent. It is not unusual for the new guy (or gal) to want to take additional emergency coverage, to an extent, while building the practice. The general terms of coverage, such as nights, weekends, and holidays, should be detailed. It should also specify how call is organized (on a seniority or equal basis). Just get a feeling for what is appropriate, and when it appears you are getting taken advantage of. A common scenario is that the senior-most, or founding partners, may often be privileged to take a disproportionately lower amount of weekend and holiday call. Although this may be standard, it is better to know earlier than later.

Vacation Policy

Most new physicians will be offered 2 weeks of vacation time, with 1 week of CME time. The second year of a contract will often increase to 3 weeks of vacation. These are typical, although variation (more or less) may be found. Negotiate with tact.

Maternity Leave

Many groups may not have an official stated policy on maternity leave. If this is relevant and appropriate to you, make sure this is discussed and included in the contract. According to the Family and Medical Leave Act of 1993, an employee is eligible for up to 12 weeks of unpaid leave during a 12-month period for the birth or adoption of a child; care for a child, spouse, or parent who is ill; and to recover from personal illness or effects from a medical treatment. This Act applies to groups with 50 or more employees or employees who have worked at least 12 months or 1,250 hours in the past 12-month period. Additional state laws may apply, and federal law states that whichever provides greater benefits in a particular situation will prevail.

Office Hours

Some, but not all, contracts will have stipulations regarding full-time and part-time hours and clinic and hospital coverage. If this exists, get an appreciation for it and if this falls within the norm for your field.

Physician Autonomy

Many, but not all, contracts should specify that although you are an employee subject to certain rules and regulations, that you also retain clinical autonomy in treating your patients.

Physician and Human Resources

Again, not all contracts spell this out, but there must be an understanding that basic office premises and equipment and clinical, as well as administrative, staff must be present and sufficiently provided in order to render services appropriately. Since the group will be adding a physician, it is important that they make provisions for your arrival. It is not unheard of to arrive, only to find a lack of facilities and employees, leaving it up to you. Not a great way to start off.

This aspect of the contract may be more important for those entering a Physician Relocation Agreement (PRA), or any situation where a third party may be involved in providing facilities and/or personnel. In this situation, an understanding of who is providing (and paying) for resources, as well as a detailed listing of what is covered, should be attached to the contract.

Sick Leave

Self-explanatory—most groups should allow for sick leave in the contract.

PART III: TERMINATION

Well, this is the aspect of the contract no one wants to think about. But just as a prenuptial agreement can make difficult proceedings a little easier, thoughtful planning here can avoid significant headaches as well as legal costs down the road.

Termination "For Cause"

Most contracts will allow for termination based on a set of certain circumstances. These are for cause items, which usually include employee shortcomings involving dishonesty, stepping outside norms of moral conduct, and indictments or convictions for felony, theft, fraud, and the like. Although it is understandable that negotiating to remove *indictments for theft* from a contract may raise a few eyebrows, it is advised to debate the inclusion of vague wording that is not specifically for cause. This includes subjective issues such as, "employee behavior that is not in the best interest of the practice." As you can correctly assume, this is wide open to interpretation and possible misuse against you.

Bilateral Rights to Terminate with Notice

Apart from the "for cause" termination, agreements may also contain language that allows for either party to terminate the agreement given a 60- to 90-day written notice, *for any reason.* During this 60- to 90-day period, fixed-salary benefits and duties will continue. If a "without cause" provision exists, it is often to your benefit to ensure that the term of notice is acceptable. Another way to look at it is this: If the contract duration is 1 year—or even 5 years—*if there is a 30 day without cause termination provision, your contract in reality could be shortened to 30 days on an instants' notice.*

Main issues surrounding termination of the contract often involve the noncompete clause. Usually, if the employee initiates the termination, a noncompete will be in force. However, if the group initiates the termination, a noncompete is usually dropped. Additionally, if the employee terminates the contract, usually within a defined period of time, certain expenses may need to be repaid to the group, including but not limited to moving expenses and signing bonuses.

If the recruit has traveled a great distance for the job, say New York to California, you may want to include a provision that prevents termination within the initial 6 months or so. This prevents an ugly surprise after uprooting yourself and your family a long distance and also allows for you to provide for contingency planning such as setting up a new practice. This can happen in situations where an institution or group experiences unexpected financial or other issues after signing you to a contract.

Noncompete Clauses

Most contracts will carry what is often called a "restrictive covenant." This essentially protects a practice from competition in the event the incoming physician leaves the group or organization. It is understandable that a practice, which may help the new physician with new referrals and practice-building, wants to prevent you from taking this goodwill across the street.

A caveat to this is that after spending time in a community, becoming established, and often developing family roots, it is not unreasonable in wanting to "set up shop" nearby. Some may look at the restrictive covenant as the price of a mistake. If the job does not work out, do you leave the city, area, or state? And for how long? And what if the job is disagreeable, but you and your family love the area? This can lead to obvious conflicts, as both are reasonable and legitimate self-interests. There are two aspects to a restrictive covenant: time and distance.

Time constraints essentially dictate the duration of the noncompete clause. Typically, 1 to 3 years are a common duration, with 1 to 2 years being more reasonable in the courts' eyes.

Distance constraints will dictate the radial distance that the noncompete clause is enforceable. A caveat of distance constraints is that not all distances are the same. What does that mean? Although a five-mile noncompete clause may not be unreasonable in a rural area, five miles may be quite significant, say in New York City, where the same radius may cover thousands of potential patients, most of whom have never been patients of the practice. In a similar vein, the noncompete distance for a pediatric cardiothoracic surgeon should not be the same as that for a general internist.

Any noncompete clause should also specify what happens upon termination. In most instances, if the physician terminates the relationship, the restrictive covenant is usually in effect. If the group terminates the physician for due cause, dissolution of the group, or relocation of the group, the restrictive covenant should generally not be enforceable.

When looking at noncompete clauses, you have to look at what you (and possibly the law) find is reasonable and legitimate based on your specialty, geography, and other relevant factors. Geographical restraint should usually cover a territory not greater than the area from which the employer draws most of its patients. As a rule, as limitations extend further in terms of time and distance, the higher the likelihood that the restrictive covenant will not be upheld by a court. This is subject to antitrust regulations, as well as a "reasonableness" standard that requires courts to consider the following:

- if the restraint is greater than necessary to protect the employer's business interests and goodwill
- if the restraint imposes undue hardship on the employee
- if the restraint is injurious to the public interest (need for medical access and care)

The clincher to a noncompete clause is a buy-out or *liquidated damages provision*, which can also on occasion serve as a penalty in case the issue goes to court. For the physician who wants to leave a group, it provides a way to go into practice nearby, as long as he or she is willing to pay for that right. For the group, it is a way to protect itself by receiving compensation for the investment it made in hiring, training, and then re-hiring another physician. A typical buy-out, which gets you out of the noncompete, can range from a years' salary, a number based on a formula, or an arbitrary amount. This can be widely variable however. To hold up in court, the amount must be based on a fair estimate of the financial expense and loss the group would incur from the physician leaving. A caveat is that if the amount is deemed excessive, it may effectively prevent a physician from leaving, causing a court to invalidate or reduce the liquidated damages.

To add to the variability, restrictive covenants vary in terms of their applicability and legal "teeth" from state to state. Some states outlaw these constraints entirely, considering such clauses as a restraint of trade. Others allow them only in the event of sale of the practice. Say that a dermatologist buys a practice in Fresno. The seller agrees not set up shop within a certain area and length of time. Although variable *(check the latest on your particular state)*, covenants not to compete are prohibited in Alabama, California, Colorado, Louisiana, Massachusetts, North Dakota, and South Dakota. Additionally, other states have reduced the scope of noncompete clauses while some courts refuse to enforce them.

In summary, the main objectives in negotiating a restrictive covenant are the following:

- Minimize the restriction to no more than 1 to 2 years. The distance should be limited to the primary practice drawing area.
- Avoid a liquidated damages clause. In many cases if the covenant is violated, the liquidated damages are upheld, and the sum is often quite large. At minimum, reduce the value of such a clause as much as possible.
- Avoid terms by which you agree to an injunction if the other party (the group or organization) alleges that you violated the provision.

Arbitration and Mediation

You may want to include a mandatory arbitration clause in your employment agreement. Arbitration is a nonjudicial proceeding that utilizes an independent, objective third party. This may be faster and more economical than utilizing a traditional court system in the event of dispute. An arbitration clause would require arbitration versus a court of law in case of dispute. There are two types of arbitration. In *nonbinding arbitration*, proceedings are held in attempt to air complaints and seek resolution. If these are not resolved, formal legal proceedings can proceed if necessary. In *binding arbitration*, both parties agree either in the contract or prior to arbitration that the results of the hearings will be binding. Furthermore, both parties forfeit the rights to pursue the dispute further in the courts. If a provision for *mediation* exists, a third party, the mediator, attempts to guide the parties to a resolution of the dispute. However, the mediator has no power to impose a resolution.

As a final note on contracts, *never sign a contract that does not fully address all the expectations and representations relating to the proposed offer.* Often you may feel that it is okay (or be made to feel so) to leave issues in the "air," and to address them as they come up. This is risky and could later pose a threat to the employment relationship over issues that could have been addressed earlier. Additionally, as the relationship continues, memories tend to fade. Each party may forget exactly what was offered or promised. *Having it in writing serves as a bedrock of information that both parties can turn to if needed.* Follow your common sense and work out all of the issues before you sign, so that you can avoid trouble down the road.

10
THE CREDENTIALING PROCESS

Every year, many physicians make the common mistake of not starting the credentialing process early enough. This often means that they cannot start practice after moving to a new area, or have a limited practice for several months secondary to limited insurance participation or licensing issues. In the best case, this can result in an unintended vacation; worse, however, are serious financial problems if your income becomes limited for a period of time.

So, how do you avoid an unpleasant situation such as that? Several months into the application process, you will likely have an idea of the region or state you intend to practice in. The sooner, the better, as you will need to initiate the credentialing process. The paperwork can be tedious and involved, and may often involve several stages and reapplications. Added to this are a need for background and reference checks, which can take time. All told, the process can last up to 6 months, so it is critical that the process is started early, as to avoid delays in starting your practice. Most importantly, no insurance will put you on their provider panel if you are not credentialed.

Medical licensing is state specific. Some requirements—including a written exam, graduation from an accredited medical school, and completion of a recognized postgraduate training program—are common to all states. Other requirements might include the length of postgraduate training, a criminal background check, an ethics and/or legal exam, and periodic competency exams.

Licensing information, including specific requirements, can be found at the Federation of State Medical Boards. The Federation of State

Medical Board's Web site (*www.fsmb.org/*) has a state-by-state directory, with links to each board's site. They can be contacted at 817-868-4000.

The Federation of State Medical Boards also runs an invaluable (fee-based) service that may help streamline the application process. The Federal Credentials Verification Service (FCVS) was established to provide a centralized, uniform process for state medical boards as well as private and governmental entities to obtain a verified, primary source record of a physician's core medical credentials. This service is designed to reduce duplication of effort by gathering, verifying, and permanently storing credentials in a centralized repository for physicians.

FCVS obtains primary source verification of medical education, postgraduate training, licensure examination history, board action history and identity. This repository of information allows an individual to establish a confidential, lifetime professional portfolio that can be forwarded at the individual's request to any interested party, including, but not limited to, state medical boards, hospitals, managed care plans, and professional societies. They can be contacted at 888-ASK-FCVS, or *www.fsmb.org*.

The next item you will need is a Drug Enforcement Administration (DEA) permit. A DEA registration is required to prescribe controlled substances. If you already have a DEA permit, make sure it's current. You'll have to submit a change of address form for your new practice location. To download an application or a change of address form, go to *www.usdoj.gov/dea* and click on "For Physicians/Registrants." Call 800-882-9539 or go to *www.deadiversion.usdoj.gov/offices_n_dirs/field-div/index.html* for a list of DEA field offices. Some states will also require a separate narcotics license.

Tired yet? Hang in there, as you'll also need a National Provider Identifier (NPI) number. This number was started as part of the government's simplification mandate, as well as to standardize health care transactions. You can apply for your NPI online or download application forms from the CMS Web site, *www.cms.hhs.gov/forms*.

The application will ask for your birth date, Social Security number, office address, specialty, and state license number. Once assigned, your NPI will never expire or change, even if you move to another state.

When you retire, or die, your number will be deactivated-not reassigned to another physician.

Finally, as a reward for getting credentialed, you'll have to take your information and apply to various insurance plans, before you start working at a practice. If you're not credentialed as a participating provider with an insurance plan, you may not be paid, and payment will go directly to the patient, or you'll receive a lower "nonparticipating" reimbursement rate. So the sooner you get on the panels of the health plans you're interested in, the better your cash flow will be.

If the practice or group you'll be working in is served by certain plans, so much the better. If you're new to a practice or to the plans in the area, you'll need to fill out a new application—which can be dozens of pages in length—and provide the necessary documentation. Most plans want a recently updated CV, copies of your state license and registration, federal and state DEA registration, and current professional liability insurance policy. A typical application requires demographic, personal, practice, and disciplinary history data.

Resist the temptation to apply to every plan, especially those that other physicians in your location have steered clear of. If you're new to a community, it may be prudent to do some research and find out what their top 10 payers are, and then apply to those plans. Medical societies keep facts and figures on the different payers, and local physicians are valuable sources of anecdotal information. Also, it wouldn't hurt to contact the benefits departments of the area's major businesses and industries and find out which insurance companies they contract with.

11

AN OVERVIEW OF SOLO PRACTICE SETUP

Starting a solo practice, whether you are fresh out of training or a seasoned physician looking to make a career shift, is a challenging task. But for all the hard work and risk, the benefits and satisfaction of managing and directing one's own practice can be quite rewarding.

Since starting a solo practice essentially entails starting a business, the intricate details of establishing a practice are beyond the scope of this text. Instead, this chapter aims to provide highlights and important issues to consider, including certain resources.

SOLO PRACTICE CONSIDERATIONS

So, who starts a solo practice? First and foremost, there should be an element of being an entrepreneur, which also entails a degree of risk tolerance. One should also appreciate needing to be an astute businessperson, as well as a clinician. Individuals who also require a degree of autonomy and control over the direction of the practice, its management, and finances will tend to do well in this regard.

Additionally, solo practice ventures require considerable time, especially over the first few years. It is important that one's family, spouse, etc, are willing to be as committed to this venture as you. A realistic appreciation of the financial aspects of the solo practice setup is also important for those starting out. Establishing a new practice, especially for those without a preexisting patient base, usually means that the practice will be operating at a loss for the first several months or greater.

Next, personality is critical, as patient and referral volume will be driven by your clinical reputation as well as personality. The latter cannot be overemphasized, as it will be up to you to shake hands with the community and establish yourself.

Finally, as the myriad of credentialing, certification, and other issues are complex, it is recommended to begin planning your solo career 1 year or longer prior to starting up.

GETTING STARTED (1 YEAR AHEAD)

Deciding on a practice location is first on the agenda. As discussed earlier in the text, several factors, including your practice specialty, will dictate the ideal location for your practice. Neurologists and cardiologists may wish to seek out retirement-type communities, whereas pediatricians may desire suburban or urban communities with a large concentration of young families. It cannot be overemphasized that the community chosen also appeals to your spouse and family.

Once a particular area is identified, a visit to the community is prudent. Meet with the local hospital and administrators, as well as potential referring physicians to understand the local medical community. Get an idea of the practices in your specialty—are they busy with long wait times, or is the competition stiff for patients? Is there an unmet subspecialty or service that you excel in? Are many of the physicians near retirement age?

As mentioned earlier, hospital administrators may be a good source of feedback for the local medical community, and what its unmet needs may be. Many hospitals may also offer financial assistance, often via Physician Recruitment Agreements (PRAs), which are covered earlier in the text. Apart from financial support, many also provide practice startup assistance in the form of practice management, advertisement, and other support services that may be invaluable in starting a practice.

Several individuals can assist in setting up a practice. Such individuals include management consultants, health care attorneys, and accountants. Although it is not necessary to have all three involved this early in the process, having initial discussions and screening individuals who you can work with will provide a degree of guidance early on. Sources for medical consultants include:

- National Association of Healthcare Consultants (www.healthcon.org). AMA's ConsultingLink (www.amaconsultinglink.com)

- Your attorney should have experience in taxation and in medical, as well as corporate, areas of practice. Your accountant similarly should have experience in medical practice financial structure and setup. A caveat to the above is to avoid individuals who also have the local hospital as a client, so as to avoid any potential conflicts of interest.

Finally, after initial meetings with the previously mentioned individuals, you will want to draft an initial business plan and budget. Whew! You're just getting started.

GETTING SERIOUS (9 MONTHS AHEAD)

Credentialing and licensing is the name of the game at this stage. You can have all your ducks in a row, but no insurance company, hospital, or state will accept you without appropriate licensure. Most licensure processes take 6 months or more, so get started early:

- Application for state medical license (if relocating)
  - o   List of state agencies and requirements
  - o   www.fsmb.org/ or 888-ASK-FCVS
- DEA registration (federal/state)
  - o   www.usdoj.gov/dea
  - o   800-882-9539
- Medicare provider number and Universal Provider Identification Number (UPIN)
  - o   www.cms.hhs.gov/providers/enrollment/contacts
  - o   877-267-2323
- Employer Identification Number (EIN)
  - o   www.irs.gov
- Medicaid provider number
  - o   www.cms.hhs.gov/medicaid/mcontact.asp

- Application for business and county licenses
  - o   Contact local chamber of commerce for details
  - o   www.chamberofcommerce.com
- Those intending to set up an in-house lab will require a CLIA certificate
  - o   www.cms.hhs.gov/clia/cliaapp.asp or 877-267-2323

The following applications can be initiated, but will likely be held up until some of the previously mentioned numbers/registration/licenses are obtained. However, it is critical to go ahead and obtain the paperwork and get started on it as early as possible.

- Insurance Plan selection and credentialing
- Hospital Staff Privileges

Finally, it will be important to scout out real estate. Important factors to consider include finding a location within reasonable distance to your population base, the local medical hospital/center, and your own home. Specific considerations for evaluating an office space include the following:

- Rent, and what it includes, such as tenant improvements (important to negotiate upfront)
- Term (including breakout and renewal policies)
- Liability issues
- Disabled access
- Utilities (who pays?)
- Noncompetition (can another physician in the same specialty open up next door?)

ESTABLISHING BENEFITS AND INSURANCE (6 MONTHS AHEAD)

Establishing appropriate benefits packages for you and your employees, as well as malpractice and disability coverage is complex. It is important to get information from your colleagues regarding insurance and casualty carriers and agents. State medical societies and local hospitals can provide information on malpractice coverage. The AMA can also provide quotes and helpful information at www.amainsure.com or 800-458-5736.

Overall, establishing appropriate coverage and benefits is where having trusted advisors, including practice management consultants, can provide invaluable guidance. The following are issues to consider:

- Evaluate malpractice coverage requirements and policies.

- Evaluate disability and workers compensation policies.

- Establish retirement/benefits plan.

- Evaluate umbrella policies (covering claims exceeding your existing coverage).

DESIGNING AND OUTFITTING YOUR PRACTICE (6 MONTHS AHEAD)

At this point, you should be close to choosing your ideal practice space. Chances are you will either be taking on a new office space or a "shell" to build out to your specifications or you will be remodeling an existing space. If you are working from scratch, hopefully you have been able to negotiate part of the "buildout" from the landlord, with the knowledge that a proper buildout will require anywhere from $50 to $100 per square foot. To follow are additional considerations:

- Interview several contractors, architects, and interior designers, depending on your needs and type of office space.

- Obtain blueprints and discuss workflow efficiency, patient and employee comfort, and aesthetic issues with the design team that you've assembled.

- Begin evaluating vendors for office furniture, clinical equipment, and supplies. For clinical and office equipment, do your research on refurbished or used equipment, as the savings can be substantial. Leasing is also an option.

- Evaluate computer and Information Technology (IT) systems. Although this may be a modest upfront expense, the headache and problems associated with converting a paper to a paperless system, not to mention retraining your staff later, may be burdensome. Starting out electronic is unquestionably the best way to start if it is financially feasible. Additionally, the Center for Medicare Services (CMS) is pushing initiatives to get physicians on Electronic Medical Records (EMRs). Higher reimbursements in certain areas for those with EMRs, lower error rates, more accurate coding, and faster insurance billing and reimbursement are among some of the potential benefits.

The main points to look for with an EMR system and IT vendor are a company that has been in the market with a long track record, and a system that is modular, or scalable. Additionally, you will want to be able to customize such a system to your practice and specialty. There are also "proprietary" systems and "open" systems; the latter are preferred as they are more easily upgradeable. Open systems are often more amenable to integration with other EMR products as well. Finally, support and upgrade availability should be included. There are hundreds of systems available, so doing your homework now can save money and headaches down the road. Do not get pushed into a fancy, complex system that you do not need early in your practice. Instead, having a system that you can grow into is much better. Having to dump a bad system and convert to another EMR can result in unneeded headaches and wasted money.

A few such systems include Logician from General Electric and Exscribe at www.exscribe.com.

- Contact the local yellow pages and phone company to establish timetables for publishing an ad, as well as obtaining a phone number. You will need to establish a business phone number, even if it is only connected to an answering machine that you check on a routine basis. A directory-listed number along with an advertisement is critical to have at the time of opening your practice.

CONTRACTING WITH INSURERS (4 MONTHS AHEAD)

This is one of the most critical aspects of planning your practice, and finding an experienced health care attorney could prove to be invaluable here. Although there will likely be many insurers in your area, it pays to be selective. Some payers have a reputation for favorable rates, methods of dispute, and arbitration management, others do not. It pays to do your homework, and the best source of this information will be the local medical society, physicians, and hospitals. Insurers that force heavily discounted fee schedules and have a reputation of excessive claim denials and rejections are best avoided.

1- to 3-year contracts are common, with negotiation periods coming up a few months prior to the contract anniversary. Shorter contracts are advisable when starting out, giving you an option to renegotiate terms or drop carriers if needed. It is critical to evaluate an insurer's fee schedule, what the reimbursement is based on, and what adjustments or "negotiated discounts" they may be able to make. You should also understand how disputes and arbitration issues are handled with the insurer.

You will want to establish a fee schedule that lists all of the commonly billed services in your practice. Fee schedules usually follow a norm for each community; many physicians opt to tie their fees to a percentage of Medicare's fee schedule. Additional information can be obtained from the state/local medical community and local physicians, or the Internet. These sources include the Center for Medicare and Medicaid Services at www.cms.hhs.gov/physicians/pfs/ or private administrators such as TrailBlazer at www.trailblazerhealth.com. Many private companies are also available to help set up a fee schedule and are readily found on the Internet.

As a final note, understand that contracting with insurers is a negotiation process, and avoid any pressure to sign a standard contract or one with which you are unfamiliar or uncomfortable. Assume that you negotiate from a position of strength, and that the insurer will need qualified, well-trained physicians such as yourself to provide care to their patients. In this vein, if you possess certain clinical skills, fellowship training, or have awards, certifications, publications, etc, it doesn't hurt to bring these points "to the table" as leverage in negotiating favorable rates or, alternatively, "carving out" special niche services that may warrant special reimbursement due to the uniqueness of the service.

ASSEMBLING YOUR TEAM (3 MONTHS AHEAD)

Having the right personnel can really make a difference between a practice that flourishes and one that runs inefficiently. Personnel and benefits packages are one of the greatest expenses of a practice. As such, starting out you will ideally need two individuals: One administrative employee to handle coding, billing, paperwork, and reception; another medical assistant or nurse to handle the clinical aspect of the practice. Interview several individuals, and screen out those who tend to have multiple, short tenures, as this may indicate instability. Definitely take the time to research and question references. Look for people with an outgoing, positive personality who will represent the "face" of your practice. Remember that your staff is always a reflection of you, and that your patients will always judge your staff as a reflection of you and your quality of work. Take your time. Start with a small but reliable core of individuals in order to keep the overhead down, and then add as the need and appropriate candidates arise. Additional issues to consider are the following:

- Educate yourself on the interview process (how to properly interview, questions to ask, and most importantly, questions you cannot ask).
- Evaluate your practice for number and type of employees required.
- Develop job/position descriptions.
- Develop job policy manuals.
- Develop office procedure manuals.
- Evaluate the local market for reasonable salary and benefit ranges.
- Research the most effective advertisement media (newspaper/Web/ local training institutions/word of mouth/community out-reach lectures and talks).

THE FINAL DETAILS (1 TO 2 MONTHS AHEAD)

This is the time to reevaluate the credentialing/licensing that you initiated several months ago. Inevitably, there may be additional questions and issues to address. In addition to this, you will need to address the following:

- Evaluate answering and transcription services.
- Evaluate phone and office communication systems.
- Choose janitorial and ancillary service companies.
- Evaluate bookkeeping, collection, banking, and payroll systems.

ALMOST THERE! (THE WEEKS AHEAD)

At this point, you are almost ready to see the fruits of your labor. You will want to make sure that you reach out to your patient population and referral sources. This includes placing announcements to the community in local print publications and postcard or other mailers to patients in the area. You will also likely want to setup a Web site. A practice brochure to give to patients on their first visit, listing services, contact information, as well as your bio, are all nice touches.

Also consider having an "open house" for the local physicians, so they can meet and greet you, the new physician, and see your facilities and get a first-hand look at the service you offer. Also, try to meet one or two new referral sources, whether they are other physicians or paramedical individuals, each week. One way is to organize a lunch meeting at their office as an introduction of you and your staff. The messages you want to convey are that you are new to the area and these are the services you provide. If you can convey to the referral sources that you are friendly, caring, and are willing to be available, that trust can lead them to refer their patients, and you will very quickly develop a loyal referral source. You should continue this practice of meeting one or two new referral sources throughout the tenure of your practice for at least the first 2 years. This will often go a long way to solidify a relationship with your referral base.

12

BASIC PRACTICE FINANCE 101

This section covers some of the basic financial terms that may be encountered, or "thrown around," when evaluating a practice or contract.

Gross Revenue:
(Gross Revenue) − (Contractual Adjustments) = **Net Revenue**

Total Expenses:
(Salaries and Benefits) + Supplies + Occupancy Expenses/Rent
+ Equipment Leases + General and Administrative Expenses
+ Depreciation and Amortization
= Total Expenses and Overhead

Gross Charges: Defined as total fees billed; an indication of productivity. Impacted by the fee schedule of the practice

Contractual Adjustments: Defined as the amount deducted from gross charges to arrive at the actual amount due to the practice. Factors in calculating the contractual adjustment include the following:

- Reimbursement rate agreed on between the practice and payor
- Discounts negotiated to reduce amounts due from patients or payor
- Write-offs, or amounts the practice has determined it will not attempt to collect
- Bad debt, or amounts that are uncollectible

Net Revenue/Collections: Defined as the amount actually collected for services provided

Collection Rate: Net revenue as a percentage of gross charges (aim for 50% or higher)

Contractual Adjustment Rate: Contractual adjustments as a percentage of gross charges

Operating Expenses: All costs resulting from daily practice operations

Overhead: The total amount of all operating expenses

Overhead Rate: The total operating expenses as a percentage of net revenue (aim for 50% or less)

Payor Mix: The percentage of the practice represented by various payor sources (Medicare, Medicaid, Managed Care, Indemnity, Self-Pay, etc.)

Individual Retirement Arrangement (IRA):   Also known as Individual Retirement Account; a type of savings account for retirement

In 2004, you could contribute up to $13,000 to a 401(k) plan—$1,000 more than you could in 2003. The limit rose to $14,000 in 2005. In 2006, the limit will rise to $15,000. If you were 50 years of age or older at year-end, you could contribute an extra $3,000 in 2004. In 2005, you can contribute $4,000; 401(k) accounts are funded generally by payroll deductions at your workplace.

1. *Deductible Traditional IRAs:* Special tax rules allow you to reduce your taxable income by your qualified contributions to your IRA. You pay tax when you make withdrawals from your IRA.

2. *Nondeductible Traditional IRAs:* Although you cannot reduce your income by the amount of your current nondeductible contributions, you do not pay tax on the earnings of your account until you make withdrawals.

3. *Roth IRAs:* You cannot deduct current contributions to a Roth IRA, but when you make qualified withdrawals from your account, you will not be taxed on the withdrawals. A Roth IRA is one of the best ways to invest money, as it can be taken out upon retirement, tax free. However, pay attention to income limits:

	Full $3000 Contribution	Reduced Contribution
Single/Head of household	Up to $95,000	$95,001–109,999
Married filing jointly	Up to $150,000	$150,001–$159,999

The new tax law makes IRAs even more attractive. The maximum annual contribution limits for traditional and Roth IRAs increase according to the following schedule:

Year	Annual Contribution Limit
2002 through 2004	$3000
2005 through 2007	$4000
2008 onward	$5000

Keogh Plan: A pension or profit-sharing plan available to self-employed individuals and their employees.

The contribution limit for self-employed Keogh plans jumped to $41,000 in 2004, up $1000 from 2003. The maximum contribution that self-employed workers can make to a Simplified Employee Pension (SEP) plan remains unchanged at the lesser of 25% of compensation, or $40,000. (The 25% limit becomes 20% if you're the owner of the business.)

IRA DEDUCTION LIMITS—2004

Filing Status	Income Level for Full Deduction	Income Level for Reduced Deduction	Income Level at Which You Receive No Deduction
Married filing jointly	Below $150,000	$150,000 to $160,000	$160,000 or more
Married filing separately	Not available	$0 to $10,000	$10,000 or more

RESOURCES

CAREER ASSISTANCE FOR PHYSICIANS

It is highly recommended to contact your individual specialty society for specific information to your area, as well as additional resources including Web-based job postings and searches that are usually at no charge for members.

Other internet sources for career assistance include:

www.epracticemanagement.org (lists of physician jobs by employers)
www.practicechoice.com (post your own CV)
www.practicelink.com (lists physician jobs by employers)
www.medbulletin.com (lists physician jobs by employers)
www.aspr.org (lists of in-house recruiters who work for employers)
www.napr.org (job posting and search organization consisting of over 400 physician recruiting firms, hospitals, medical groups, and individuals)

COMPENSATION INFORMATION

American Medical Association

1-800-621-8335

Center for Healthcare Industry Performance Studies

301-458-4636

American Medical Group Association

1422 Duke St.
Alexandria, VA 22314
703-838-0033
www.amga.org

The AMGA exclusively surveys physicians in large multispecialty groups. Its 2000 Medical Group Compensation & Productivity Survey costs $175 for members and $250 for nonmembers.

The Healthcare Group
Meetinghouse Business Center
140 West Germantown Pike, Suite 200
Plymouth Meeting, PA 19462
800-473-0032
www.healthcaregroup.com
Produces an annual Physician Starting Salary Survey. Free upon registering on website.

Medical Economics magazine
5 Paragon Drive
Montvale, NJ 07645
www.memag.com
The magazine publishes the results of its annual Continuing Survey, a series of reports on physicians' practice incomes, fees and reimbursements, etc.

Medical Group Management Association
104 Inverness Terrace East
Englewood, CO 80112
877-275-6462
www.mgma.com
The MGMA gathers data from its member organizations, which represent groups of all sizes, for its annual MGMA Physician Compensation and Production Survey. Buy the survey online or by calling 877.275.6462 ext 888. The cost is $225 for MGMA members, $320 for affiliates, $480 for nonmembers. A truncated version is available free on the website.

Cejka and Company
222 South Central Ave, Suite 400
St. Louis, MO 63105
314-726-1603 (800-678-7858)
www.cejka.com
This health care consulting and search firm does a biennial Physician Executive Compensation Survey in collaboration with the American

College of Physician Executives. A free summary of the survey is available at the Compensation section of their Web site.

CONTRACT NEGOTIATIONS

Organizations

American Medical Association
515 North State St.
Chicago, IL 60610
312-464-5000
www.ama-assn.org
For help with your employment agreement, consult the AMA's "Annotated Model Physician Employment Agreement," and "Contracts: What You Need to Know," both available at *www.ama-assn.org/ama/priv/category/2207.html* (for AMA members). To request a free hard copy of the Annotated Model Physician Employment Agreement, AMA members can call 312-464-4978.

AMA ConsultingLink
(Provided by AMA subsidiaries)
800-366-6968
www.amaconsultinglink.com (Click on Consultants & Attorneys.)
If you're looking for legal assistance, try AMA ConsultingLink, which will provide for free the names of two or three health care attorneys, as well as other business consultants, in your area.

Books

Evaluating and Negotiating Compensation Arrangements. Chicago: American Medical Association; 2000.

The Physician's Resume and Cover Letter Workbook. Chicago: American Medical Association; 2000.

The Physician in Transition: Managing the Job Interview. Chicago: American Medical Association; 2000.

Assessing Your Career Options. Chicago: American Medical Association; 2000.

Starting a Medical Practice. Chicago: American Medical Association; 2000.

Financial Management of the Medical Practice. Chicago: American Medical Association; 2000.

Assessing the Value of the Medical Practice. Chicago: American Medical Association; 2000.

Buying, Selling, and Owning the Medical Practice. Chicago: American Medical Association; 2000.

Hirsh, JD.B. *How to Negotiate a Physician's Employment Contract*. Chicago/Dallas: American Medical Association and Texas Medical Association; 1999.

Babitsky, S., Mangraviti. J J. *The Successful Physician Negotiatior: How to Get What You Deserve*. Tampa: American College of Physician Executives;1999.

Kaufman, R. *The Business Side of Medicine: A Survival Primer for Medical Students and Residents*. Tampa: American College of Physician Executives; 1999.

Double, D.L. *The Physician in Transition: Managing the Job Interview*. Chicago: American Medical Association, 1997.

Kashani, J.H., Allan, W.D., Kelly, K. *The Physician's Job-Search Rx: Marketing Yourself for the Position You Want*. New York: John Wiley & Sons, 1998.

Todd, M.K. *Physician Employment Contract Handbook*. New York: McGraw-Hill and the Medical Group Management Association, 1999.

Hekman, K.M. (ed.). *Physician Compensation, Models for Aligning Financial Goals and Incentives*. New York: McGraw-Hill, 2000.

Medical Economics. You'll find the magazine's new Career Center at the magazine's home page (*www.memag.com*). You can search or post available physician jobs, obtain one-on-one career counseling, and post your CV.

The New England Journal of Medicine (*www.nejm.org/careerlinks*) gives registered members the option to receive e-mail alerts of new job openings before they're listed online or in print, or to access them as they become available. Also provides links to some recruitment firms and related articles on careers.

Starting Your Own Practice

American Medical Association and American Academy of Family Physicians: *Starting a Medical Practice*; order at *www.amapress.org* or at 1 800-621-8335

American Academy of Family Physicians: *On Your Own: Starting a Medical Practice From the Ground Up*; order at *www.aafp.org/x19744.xml* or at 1 800-944-0000

LICENSURE AND CERTIFICATION

- Application for state medical license (if relocating)
  - o List of state agencies and requirements
  - o *www.fsmb.org* or 888-ASK-FCVS
- DEA registration (federal/state)
  - o *www.usdoj.gov/dea*
  - o 800-882-9539
- Medicare provider number and Universal Provider Identification Number (UPIN)
  - o www.cms.hhs.gov/providers/enrollment/contacts
  - o 877-267-2323
- Employer Identification Number (EIN)
  - o *www.irs.gov*
- Medicaid provider number
  - o *www.cms.hhs.gov/medicaid/mcontact.asp*
- Application for business and county licenses
  - o Contact local chamber of commerce for details
  - o *www.chamberofcommerce.com*
- Clinical Laboratory Improvement Amendments (CLIA) certificate
  - o *www.cms.hhs.gov/clia/cliaapp.asp* or 877-267-2323

RECRUITERS

Cejka Search
www.cejkasearch.com
Offers a list of job openings, a career development library, and the opportunity for a live consultation with a career counselor. You can also post legal questions to an attorney.

J & C Nationwide
www.jcnationwide.com
Formerly Jackson & Coker and Nationwide Medical Services, the firm lists openings for permanent and locum tenens positions, along with articles on career basics.

Merritt, Hawkins & Associates
www.merritthawkins.com
This large physician recruitment company in Irving, TX, lists job openings, best places to live, housing information, etc, plus related links.

National Association of Physician Recruiters
World Job Bank
www.napr.org
Posts permanent and locum tenens positions available in the US as well as in Canada, Guam, Puerto Rico, and the Virgin Islands. The NAPR's membership includes physician recruitment firms, hospitals, medical groups, individuals, and vendor organizations.

Pederson & Freedman
ilw.com
Includes links to medical journals with job ads, recruitment firms/organizations, and Internet employment advertising. Intended as a resource for foreign physicians but useful for all doctors.

Trapani & Associates
www.webdoc.com
This New Orleans-based firm offers an integrated online network system, database of over 700 practice opportunities by specialty, and employment-related articles.

Comphealth
www.comphealth.com
Comphealth another major recruitment firm, lists practice and locum tenens opportunities and offers a career guide with articles on career basics.

Worldwide Medical Services
www.wwmedical.com
The site provides job listings for locum tenens and permanent placement, along with an area for client registration.

PHYSICIAN COMPENSATION GUIDE

Things get a bit dicey when it comes to pinning down physician compensation, leading to usage of the word *guide*. First, it is important to know that these are *compensation* guides, and not *salary* guides. What's the difference? Salary is the upfront dollar figure, or wages paid on a regular basis, while compensation comprises retirement benefits, health insurance, bonuses, and the like. So, use the tables that follow with a good dose of diligence, understanding that local demand, geography, and individual factors will play a large role in determining your final compensation.

PHYSICIAN COMPENSATION GUIDE BY SPECIALTY

SPECIALTY	YEARS 1–2	3	ESTABLISHED/HIGH
Allergy/Immunology	$150,000	$220,000	$490,000
Anesthesiology: Pediatrics	$280,000	$310,000	$380,000
Anesthesiology: General	$210,000	$275,000	$450,000
Anesthesiology: Pain Management	$315,000	$370,000	$650,000
Cardiology: Invasive	$250,000	$400,000	$650,000
Cardiology: Interventional	$290,000	$470,000	$800,000
Cardiology: Noninvasive	$225,000	$350,000	$600,000
Critical Care	$150,000	$220,000	$320,000
Dermatology	$180,000	$250,000	$375,000
Emergency Medicine	$170,000	$220,000	$300,000
Endocrinology	$145,000	$180,000	$240,000
FP (with OB)	$130,000	$175,000	$240,000
FP (w/o OB)	$120,000	$150,000	$220,000
FP—Sports Medicine	$150,000	$210,000	$360,000
FP—Urgent Care	$130,000	$198,000	$299,000
Gastroenterology	$210,000	$300,000	$500,000
Hematology/Oncology	$180,000	$240,000	$680,000

(Continued)

PHYSICIAN COMPENSATION GUIDE BY SPECIALTY (*CONTINUED*)

SPECIALTY	YEARS 1–2	>3	ESTABLISHED/HIGH
Infectious Disease	$140,000	$180,000	$270,000
Internal Medicine	$125,000	$160,000	$220,000
IM (Hospitalist)	$150,000	$170,000	$250,000
Medicine/Pediatrics	$140,000	$170,000	$270,000
Medical Oncology	$200,000	$260,000	$450,000
Neonatal Medicine	$150,000	$210,000	$380,000
Nephrology	$160,000	$220,000	$425,000
Neurology	$150,000	$200,000	$340,000
Obstetrics/Gynecology	$200,000	$240,000	$380,000
Gynecology	$180,000	$220,000	$360,000
Maternal/Fetal Medicine	$280,000	$320,000	$610,000
Occupational Medicine	$140,000	$180,000	$290,000
Ophthalmology	$175,000	$250,000	$450,000
Ophthalmology Retina	$280,000	$470,000	$720,000
Orthopedic Surgery	$250,000	$350,000	$670,000
ORS—Foot & Ankle	$230,000	$390,000	$790,000
ORS—Hand & Upper Extremities	$290,000	$380,000	$770,000
ORS—Hip & Joint Replacement	$330,000	$430,000	$715,000
ORS—Spine Surgery	$325,000	$550,000	$1,400,000
ORS—Sports Medicine	$260,000	$480,000	$760,000
Otorhinolaryngology	$200,000	$300,000	$520,000
Pathology	$170,000	$260,000	$610,000
Pediatrics	$125,000	$165,000	$270,000
Pediatrics–Cardiology	$150,000	$280,000	$600,000
Pediatrics–Critical Care	$170,000	$200,000	$390,000
Pediatrics–Hematology/Oncology	$180,000	$200,000	$250,000
Pediatrics–Neurology	$160,000	$180,000	$360,000
Pediatrics–Hematology/Oncology	$180,000	$200,000	$250,000
Pediatrics–Neurology	$160,000	$180,000	$360,000
Physiatry	$160,000	$210,000	$310,000
Podiatry	$120,000	$170,000	$290,000
Psychiatry	$135,000	$170,000	$240,000
Psychiatry–Child and Adolescent	$150,000	$180,000	$265,000
Pulmonary Medicine + Critical Care	$215,000	$280,000	$420,000
Radiation Oncology	$220,000	$380,000	$780,000
Radiology (Diagnostic)	$200,000	$350,000	$900,000
Radiology (Interventional)	$260,000	$400,000	$530,000
Rheumatology	$140,000	$180,000	$300,000
Surgery–General	$200,000	$270,000	$450,000
Surgery–Cardiovascular	$300,000	$500,000	$800,000
Surgery–Neurological	$320,000	$420,000	$900,000
Surgery–Plastic	$225,000	$350,000	$800,000
Surgery—Vascular	$245,000	$330,000	$530,000
Urology	$220,000	$300,000	$500,000

APPENDIX 3

PHYSICIAN COMPENSATION AND BENEFITS WORKSHEET

Physician Compensation and Benefits Worksheet: This reflects factors that should be taken into consideration in determining your salary, benefits, and overall physician compensation. It is important to fill this out for each of your serious job considerations, and then compare the pros and cons of each offer.

Questions:	Yes/No	Benefits or Other Factors	Cost to You	Salary or Benefit Value per annum
What is the base pay offered, and how does it compare to your expected salary range?			$	$
If the salary is at the high end of the range, are there expenses you will assume yourself from the benefits listed below?		Use the "Cost to You" column.		
Are there factors to offset a low salary, and do they have a monetary value or other value to you?		Calculate yearly values of benefits and record in the far column.		

(Continued)

Questions:	Yes/No	Benefits or Other Factors	Cost to You	Salary or Benefit Value per annum
Are bonuses offered, annual or other?		Expected amount?		
How are the above bonuses determined?				
When are the above bonuses paid?				
Is there partnership potential and when?				
Can you accept other income from other sources such as speaking engagements, authorships, moon-lighting, etc.?				
Is there a restrictive covenant?		Length of time and/or geo-graphic area?		
Benefits: Assign a yearly value				
FICA/Medicare paid?				
Health insurance? Portion paid?		Cost to you?		
Life insurance (face value)?		Cost to you?		
Dental insurance?		Cost to you?		
Short-term disability?		Cost to you? Duration? % of pay?		
Long-term disability?		Cost to you? Duration? % of pay?		

(Continued)

Questions:	Yes/No	Benefits or Other Factors	Cost to You	Salary or Benefit Value per annum
Pension plan?		Defined Benefit? Defined Contribution? Vesting schedule?		
401(K) or other retirement savings?		Maximum contribution? Before or after tax? Vesting schedule?		
Company match: Profit sharing?		How much?		
Company match: Student loans?		How much?		
Professional dues and licensing?		Record both those paid for by your employer and those you will need to assume yourself.		
Malpractice insurance?		Coverage limitations individual and aggregate? Record any cost to yourself.		
Tail coverage?				
CME allowance?				
Auto allowance?				
Auto insurance?				
Cellular phone expenses?				
Parking?				

(Continued)

Questions:	Yes/No	Benefits or Other Factors	Cost to You	Salary or Benefit Value per annum
Other benefits (record value):		Number of days and amount.		
Vacation pay?				
Sick pay?				
CME/professional development?				
Family leave?				
Nonfinancial benefits:				
Office physical environment?				
Practice culture?				
Other physicians?				
Staff?				
Commute?				
Cost of living?		This may decrease or increase the value of an offer significantly.		
Desirability of location with regard to your lifestyle, family, recreational activities and/or career advancement.				
Total yearly cost to you for benefits:			−$	
Total yearly value of salary and benefits:				+$
Total Compensation:				$$

INDEX

Page numbers followed by italic *f* or *t* indicate figures or tables, respectively.

Academic applications, 37–38, 40f–43f
Academic practice, 23, 32–35
AMA (American Medical Association), 121, 123
AMA ConsultingLink, 123
AMGA (American Medical Group Association), 121–122
Ancillary revenue streams, 74
Ancillary services, 115
Applications
    academic, 37–38, 40f–43f
    private practice, 38, 44f–45f
    for solo practice setup, 110
Arbitration and mediation, 102
Arts and culture, in top cities, 4t, 5t
Assistance, career, for physicians, 121
Attorney, services of, 84

Balance sheet, P&L statements and, 81
Banking system, 115
Benefits
    fringe, 91–92
    insurance and, 110–111
    of PRAs, 65
    worksheet for, 132
Bilateral rights, to terminate with notice, 99
Bonuses
    collection-based, 72–73
    compensation package relating to, 72–73, 86–87
    production-based, 73, 87
    RVU-based, 73
    sign-on incentive, 86

Bookkeeping system, 115
Budgets, operating and capital, 81, 109
Business plan, 109
Buy-in/buy-out formula, 94–96
Buy-out or liquidated damages provision, 101

Call coverage, 96
Candidate, profile of, 3–24
    finances in, 16
    marital and family status in, 3, 16
    two-physician families' needs in, 16
Career assistance, for physicians, 121
Career search, planning for, July-to-June timeframe in, 2
Cause, for termination, 98
Cejka and Company, 122–123, 125
Center for Healthcare Industry Performance Studies, 121
Centers for Medicare & Medicaid Services. *See* CMS
Cities, top overall
    in arts and culture, 4t, 5t
    in climate, 4t
    in cost of living, 4t, 5t
    in economy and jobs, 4t
    in education, 4t
    in job growth, 5t
    list for, 19–23
    in nightlife, 5t
    in number of singles, 5t
Claims-made policy, 90
Climate, in top cities, 4t
CMS (Centers for Medicare & Medicaid Services), 72

Collection rate, 118
Collection system, 115
Collection-based bonuses, 72–73
Collections/net revenue, 117
Communication services, 115
Compensation, benefits worksheet
    and, 132
Compensation guide, 127–128
Compensation package
    ancillary revenue streams relating
        to, 74
    bonuses as part of, 72–73
    fixed salary as, 71
    formula-based, 71
    group or physician net income,
        based on, 70–71
    information resources for,
        121–123
    negotiations for, 63–64
    productivity, based on, 70
    RVU-based salary as, 72
    salary v., 63
    taxes relating to, 73–74
Comphealth, 126
Contract, negotiations for
    attorney's services relating to, 84
    compensation
        bonus, 86–87
        disability insurance, 88–89
        fringe benefits, 91–92
        health insurance, 88
        insurance coverage, 88
        life insurance, 90
        malpractice insurance and tail
            coverage, 89–90
        retirement or pension plans, 91
        salary, 86
    pitfalls of
        "attach it," 85
        "don't assume," 85
        "get it in writing," 85
        "negotiate, negotiate,
            negotiate," 85
        "take time," 85

process, understanding of, 83–86
resources for, 123–124
termination
    arbitration and mediation, 102
    bilateral rights to terminate with
        notice, 99
    for cause, 98
    noncompete clauses, 99–101
terms of employment
    call coverage, 96
    duration, 93
    financing, 96
    maternity leave, 96
    no partnership opportunity, 96
    office hours, 97
    partnership and buy-in/buy-out
        formula, 94–96
    physician and human resources,
        97–98
    physician autonomy, 97
    physician's duties, scope of,
        93–94
    sick leave, 98
    vacation policy, 97
Contractual adjustment rate, 118
Contractual adjustments, 117
Cost of living
    salary range v., 16
    in top cities, 4t, 5t
Cover letter, for CV, 37, 39f
Credentialing, process of
    insurance relating to, 104
    licensing information, 103–104,
        109–110, 114
    NPI number, 104
    permits, 104
Culture. See arts and culture,
        in top cities
CV (curriculum vitae), 105
    for academic applications, 37–38,
        40f–43f
    cover letter for, 37, 39f
    for private practice applications,
        38, 44f–45f

DEA (Drug Enforcement
    Administration) permit,
    104–105
Deductible traditional IRA, 118–119
Department of Health and Human
    Services, 66
Direct costs, 75
Disability insurance, 88–89
    individual, group v., 89
    "own occupation" relating to, 88–89
    taxes relating to, 88
Distance constraints, 100
Drug Enforcement Administration.
    See DEA
Dues, 92
Duties, of physicians, 93–94

Economy and jobs, in top cities, 4t
Education, in top cities, 4t
Employment, terms of, 93–98
Equal assessment, 75
Expenses
    direct costs, 75
    equal assessment, 75
    indirect costs, 75
    operating, 118
    percentage of productivity relating
        to, 75
    total, 117

FCVS (Federal Credentials
    Verification Service), 104
Federation of State Medical Boards
    (www.fsmb.org/), 103–104
Finances, in candidate profile, 16
Financial analysis, of group, 61–62
    information included in
        anticipated major projects
            and costs, 79
        balance sheet and P&L
            statements, 81
        current income distribution
            plan, 79
        management, 80

operating and capital budgets, 81
outlook and goals, 79
overhead-to-revenue ratio, 78
payor mix for last 3 to 5 years,
    79–80
physician productivity
    summary, 81
practice debt, 81
provider contracts, 80
realistic production rate, 79
receivables history, 81
retirement policy, 80
Financial support, 108
Financial terms, 117–119
Financing, 96
Fixed salary, 71
Formula-based compensation
    package, 71
Fringe benefits
    dues and licenses, 92
    housing and related matters, 91–92
    moving, 91
    outside income policy, 92
    student loan payments, 92
    vacation and sick leave, 92

Goals, 16–18, 79
Government practice, 23, 36
Gross charges, 117
Gross revenue, 117
Group net income, 70–71

Health insurance, 88
The Healthcare Group, 122
Home, four bedroom, average cost
    of, 6–15t
Housing, 91–92
http://costoflivingwizard.salary.com, 18
http://money.cnn.com/real_estate/
    best_places, 18
http://www.bestplaces.net/fybp/, 18
http://www.relocationessentials.com/
    tools/crime/crime.asp, 18
Human resources, 97–98

Income, 16–17. *See also* group net
     income; net income guarantee;
     outside income policy
Income distribution plan, 79
Income loan, 69–70
Indirect costs, 75
Individual disability insurance, 89
Individual Retirement Account/
     Arrangement. *See* IRA
Insurance, 104, 110–111. *See also*
     Specific insurance headings
Insurance coverage, 88
Interview, evaluation process of
  financial analysis of group, 61–62
  impression as part of, 53–55
     personality conflicts relating
        to, 54
     questions relating to, 54–55
  indepth questions of group, 55–60
  work surroundings as part of
     community, 61
     daily operations, 61
     environment, 60
     resources, 60–61
IRA (Individual Retirement Account).
     See also Keogh Plan
  contribution limits, 119
  deductible traditional, 118–119
  deduction limits, 119
  nondeductible traditional,
     118–119
  Roth, 118–119

J & C Nationwide, 125
Janitorial and ancillary services, 115
Job growth, in top cities, 5*t*
Job search, sources for
  pharmaceutical representatives, 58
  recruiters, 59–61
  residents, 57
  staff physicians, 58
  time relating to, 57
Jobs, in top cities, 4*t*

Keogh Plan, 119. *See also* IRA

Licensing information, 92, 103–104,
     125. *See also* credentialing,
     process of
Life insurance, 90
Liquidated damages provision, 101
Location, 108. *See also* cities, top
     overall
  considerations of
     long-term goals, 16–18
     salary, income v., 16–17
     short-term goals, 16–18
  pitfalls of, 16–18
  rank lists for, 17–18
  web sites relating to, 18
Locum tenens, 23
Long-term goals, 16–18

Malpractice insurance and tail
     coverage
  claims-made policy, 90
  occurrence policy, 89–90
Managed care company, 23
Management, of group, 80
Marital and family status, in
     candidate profile, 3, 16
Maternity leave, 96
Mediation. *See* arbitration and
     mediation
Medical consultants, 108–09
Medical Economics, 122
Merritt, Hawkins & Associates, 126
MGMA (Medical Group
     Management Association),
     122
Moving, 91
MSG (multispecialty group practice),
     23–36, 28*f*

National Association of Physician
     Recruiters, 126
National Provider Identifier. *See* NPI

Negotiations
   for compensation package, 63–64
   for contract (*See* contract,
      negotiations for)
Net income, 70–71
Net income guarantee, 67–68
Net revenue/collections, 117
Nightlife, in top cities, 5t
"no partnership opportunity," 96
Noncompete clauses
   buy-out or liquidated damages
      provision, 101
   distance constraints, 100
   "reasonableness" standard relating
      to, 100
   restrictive covenant, 99–101
   time constraints, 100
Nondeductible traditional IRA, 118–119
NPI (National Provider Identifier)
   number, 104

Occurrence policy, 89–90
Office hours, 97
Operating expenses, 118
Outside income policy, 92
Overhead rate, 118
Overhead-to-revenue ratio, 78
"Own occupation," disability
   insurance relating to, 88–89

Partnership, buy-in/buy-out formula
   and, 94–96
Payor mix, 79–80, 118
Payroll system, 115
Pederson & Freedman, 126
Pension plans, 91. *See also*
   retirement or pension plans
Percentage of productivity, 75
Permits, 104
Personality conflicts, 54
Pharmaceutical representatives, 58
Phone, communication services
   and, 115

Physician autonomy, 97
Physician productivity summary, 81
Physician Recruitment Agreements.
   See PRAs
Physicians. *See also* two-physician
   families' needs
   career assistance for, 121
   duties of, 93–94
   human resources and, 97–98
   net income of, 70–71
   staff for, 58
P&L statements, 81
Practice debt, 81
Practice, designing and outfitting of,
   111–112
Practice, ideal, types of. *See also* solo
   practice setup
   academic, 23
      elements of, 32–35
      pros and cons of, 35
   government, 23
      pros and cons of, 36
   locum tenens, 23
      pros and cons of, 36
   managed care company, 23
   MSG, 23
      elements of, 31–32
      pros and cons of, 32
   single specialty, large group, 23
      advantages and disadvantages of,
      29–30
      pros and cons of, 30–31
   single specialty, small group, 23
      elements of, 27–28, 28f
      pros and cons of, 28
   solo practitioner, 23
      factors of, 23–25
      issues relating to, 24
      pros and cons of, 25
      resources for, 24
   solo practitioner, joining of, 23
      issues relating to, 26
      pros and cons of, 27

PRAs (Physician Recruitment
     Agreements), 24, 64–70
  benefits of, 65
  legalities relating to, 66–67
  salary provided by
     income loan as, 69–70
     net income guarantee as, 67–68
Private practice applications, 38,
     44f–45f
Production rate, 79
Productivity
  bonuses based on, 73, 87
  compensation package based on, 70
  salary based on, 86
Profile. See candidate, profile of
Provider contracts, 80

Rank lists, for locations, 17–18
Real estate, 110
"Reasonableness" standard, 100
Receivables history, 81
Recruiters, 59–61
Referral source, development of, 115
Relative value unit. See RVU
Residents, 57
Resources
  career assistance for physicians, 121
  compensation information, 121–123
  contract negotiations, 123–124
  licensure and certification, 125
  recruiters, 125–126
  for solo practitioner, 24
  for work surroundings, 60–61
Restrictive covenant, 99–101
Resume. See CV (curriculum vitae)
Retirement or pension plans, 80, 91.
     See also IRA
Roth IRA, 118–119
RVU (relative value unit), 72
RVU-based bonuses, 73
RVU-based salary, 72
Salary, 16–17, 86. See also
     compensation package; PRAs

Short-term goals, 16–18
Sick leave, 92, 98
Sign-on incentive bonus, 86
Single specialty practice, 23, 27–31, 28f
Singles, numbers of, in top cities, 5t
Solo practice setup
  1–2 months ahead
     bookkeeping, collection, banking,
        payroll systems, 115
     credentialing/licensing,
        reevaluation of, 114
     janitorial and ancillary
        services, 115
     phone and communication
        services, evaluation of, 115
     transcription services, evaluation
        of, 115
  3 months ahead
     team, assembling of, 114
  4 months ahead
     insurers, contracting with,
        112–113
  6 months ahead
     benefits and insurance, 110–111
     designing and outfitting practice,
        111–112
  considerations for, 107–108
  getting serious (9 months ahead)
     applications, 110
     credentialing and licensing,
        109–110
     real estate, 110
  getting started (1 year ahead),
        108–109
     business plan and budget, 109
     financial support, 108
     location, 108
     medical consultants, 108–09
  weeks ahead
     announcements, open house, 115
     referral source, development
        of, 115
     web site, 115

Solo practitioner, 23
    factors of, 23–25
    issues relating to, 24, 26
    pros and cons of, 25, 27
    resources for, 24
Staff, for physicians, 58
Staff physicians, 58
Student loan payments, 92

Tail coverage. *See* malpractice
        insurance and tail coverage
Taxes
    compensation package relating to,
        73–74
    disability insurance relating to, 88

Termination, 98–102
Terms, of employment, 93–98
Time constraints, 100
Total expenses, 117
Transcription services, 115
Trapani & Associates, 126
Two-physician families' needs, 16

Vacation policy, 92, 97

Web sites, 103–104, 121
    for locations, 18
    for solo practice, 115
Work surroundings, 60–61
Worldwide Medical Services, 126